# MY PASTA RECIPES 2022

## AUTHENTIC ITALIAN RECIPES MADE EASY

GIULIO PATRIZI

# TABLE OF CONTENTS

# *Ziti with Spinach and Ricotta*

## *Ziti con Spinaci e Ricotta*

**Makes 4 to 6 servings**

*Spinach, ricotta, and Parmigiano-Reggiano are a typical stuffing for ravioli in Emilia-Romagna and many other regions. In this recipe, the filling for fresh pasta becomes the sauce for dried pasta. The flavors are similar, but the method is much easier for every day. Chopped cooked broccoli can stand in for the spinach if you like.*

1½ pounds spinach, tough stems removed

4 tablespoons unsalted butter

1 medium onion, finely chopped

Salt

1 pound ziti or penne

1 cup whole or part-skim ricotta, at room temperature

½ cup freshly grated Parmigiano-Reggiano

Freshly ground black pepper

**1.** Put the spinach in a large pot over medium heat with $^{1}/_{4}$ cup water. Cover and cook for 2 to 3 minutes or until wilted and tender. Drain and cool. Wrap the spinach in a lint-free cloth and squeeze out as much water as possible. Finely chop the spinach.

**2.** In a large saucepan, melt the butter over medium-low heat. Add the onion and cook until tender and golden, about 10 minutes. Add the chopped spinach and cook, stirring, until the spinach is heated through, 3 to 4 minutes. Add salt to taste

**3.** Bring at least 4 quarts of water to a boil in a large pot. Add 2 tablespoons of salt, then the pasta. Stir well. Cook over high heat, stirring frequently, until the pasta is al dente, tender yet still firm to the bite. Drain the pasta, reserving some of the cooking water.

**4.** In a large heated serving bowl, toss the pasta with the spinach, ricotta, and cheese. Add a little of the cooking water if the pasta seems dry. Sprinkle with freshly ground black pepper and serve immediately.

# *Rigatoni with Four Cheeses*

## *Rigatoni ai Quattro Formaggi*

**Makes 4 to 6 servings**

*The four cheeses suggested below are just a suggestion. Use whatever you have on hand, even pieces that are a little dried out are fine when grated. I can't think of any cheese that does not go well with pasta. I have eaten versions of this pasta in Rome, Tuscany, and Naples, and I suspect it is the kind of thing that cooks throw together whenever they have small amounts of a variety of cheeses.*

1 pound rigatoni, ziti, or fusilli

Salt

6 tablespoons unsalted butter, melted

½ cup shredded Fontina Valle d'Aosta

½ cup shredded fresh mozzarella

½ cup shredded Gruyere or Emmenthal

¾ cup freshly grated Parmigiano-Reggiano

Freshly ground black pepper

**1.** Bring at least 4 quarts of water to a boil in a large pot. Add 2 tablespoons of salt, then the pasta. Stir well. Cook over high heat, stirring frequently, until the pasta is al dente, tender but still firm to the bite. Drain the pasta, reserving some of the cooking water.

**2.** In a large heated serving bowl, toss the pasta with the butter. Add the cheeses and a couple of tablespoons of the pasta water. Toss until the cheese is melted. Sprinkle with black pepper and serve immediately.

# *Linguine with Creamy Nut Sauce*

## *Linguine con Salsa di Noci*

**Makes 4 to 6 servings**

*My friend Pauline Wasserman came across this recipe while traveling in Piedmont and gave it to me some years ago. The nuts give the pasta a rich flavor, while the ricotta keeps it creamy and moist. I serve it with dolcetto, a light, dry red wine from Piedmont.*

½ cup walnuts

2 tablespoons pine nuts

4 tablespoons unsalted butter

1 small garlic clove, very finely chopped

1 tablespoon chopped fresh flat-leaf parsley

¼ cup whole or part-skim ricotta, mascarpone, or heavy cream

Salt

1 pound linguine

½ cup freshly grated Parmigiano-Reggiano

1. Place the walnuts and pine nuts in a food processor or blender. Grind the nuts just until fine. (Don't overprocess into a paste.)

2. In a medium skillet, melt the butter over medium heat. Add the garlic and parsley and cook 1 minute. Stir in the ground nuts and ricotta. Stir to blend and heat through.

3. Meanwhile, bring about 4 quarts of water to a boil in a large pot. Add 2 tablespoons of salt, then the pasta, gently pushing it down until the pasta is completely covered with water. Stir well. Cook, stirring often, until the pasta is al dente, tender yet still firm to the bite. Set aside some of the cooking water. Drain the pasta.

4. In a large heated serving bowl, toss the pasta with the sauce and grated cheese. Add a little of the cooking water if the pasta seems dry. Serve immediately.

# *Bow Ties with Amaretti*

## *Farfalle con gli Amaretti*

**Makes 4 to 6 servings**

*One of the specialties of Lombardy is fresh egg pasta stuffed with winter squash and crushed* amaretti, *crunchy almond cookies (Winter Squash Ravioli with Butter and Almonds). Bathed in melted butter and sprinkled with salty and nutty Parmigiano, the combination of flavors is most unusual and unforgettable. The waiter at a little trattoria in Cremona told me that this simple recipe made with dried pasta was inspired by that elaborate dish.*

*If your raisins are on the dry side, plump them by dropping them into the boiling pasta water just before draining.*

Salt

1 pound farfalle

1 stick unsalted butter, melted

12 to 16 amaretti cookies, crushed (about ½ cup crumbs)

⅓ cup golden raisins

1 cup grated Parmigiano-Reggiano

**1.** Bring at least 4 quarts of water to a boil in a large pot. Add 2 tablespoons of salt, then the pasta. Stir well. Cook over high heat, stirring frequently, until the pasta is al dente, tender yet still firm to the bite. Set aside some of the cooking water. Drain the pasta.

**2.** Place the butter in a large warm serving bowl. Add the pasta and toss it with the cookie crumbs and raisins. Add the cheese and toss again. Add a little of the cooking water if the pasta seems dry. Serve hot.

# *Spaghetti with Fried Eggs, Salerno Style*

## *Spaghetti con l'Uuovo Fritto alla Salernitana*

**Makes 2 servings**

*Though I had heard about this recipe from the Naples area, I never tried making it until one day when I thought I had nothing in the house to cook for myself and my husband. It is simple and comforting and could even be served for brunch. The eggs should be cooked until the whites are set but the yolks are still soft. The ingredients for this recipe will serve two, but you can double or triple them as needed.*

4 ounces spaghetti or linguine

Salt

2 tablespoons olive oil

4 eggs

½ cup freshly grated Pecorino Romano

Freshly ground black pepper

**1.** Bring at least 4 quarts of water to a boil in a large pot. Add 2 tablespoons of the salt, then the pasta, gently pushing it down until the pasta is completely covered with water. Stir well. Cook over high heat, stirring frequently.

**2.** Heat the oil in a large skillet over medium heat. Add the eggs, sprinkling them with salt and pepper. Cook until the whites are just set and the yolks are still soft.

**3.** Drain the pasta, reserving some of the cooking water. Toss the pasta with the cheese and 2 to 3 tablespoons of the water.

**4.** Divide the pasta between 2 serving dishes. Top each with two eggs and serve immediately.

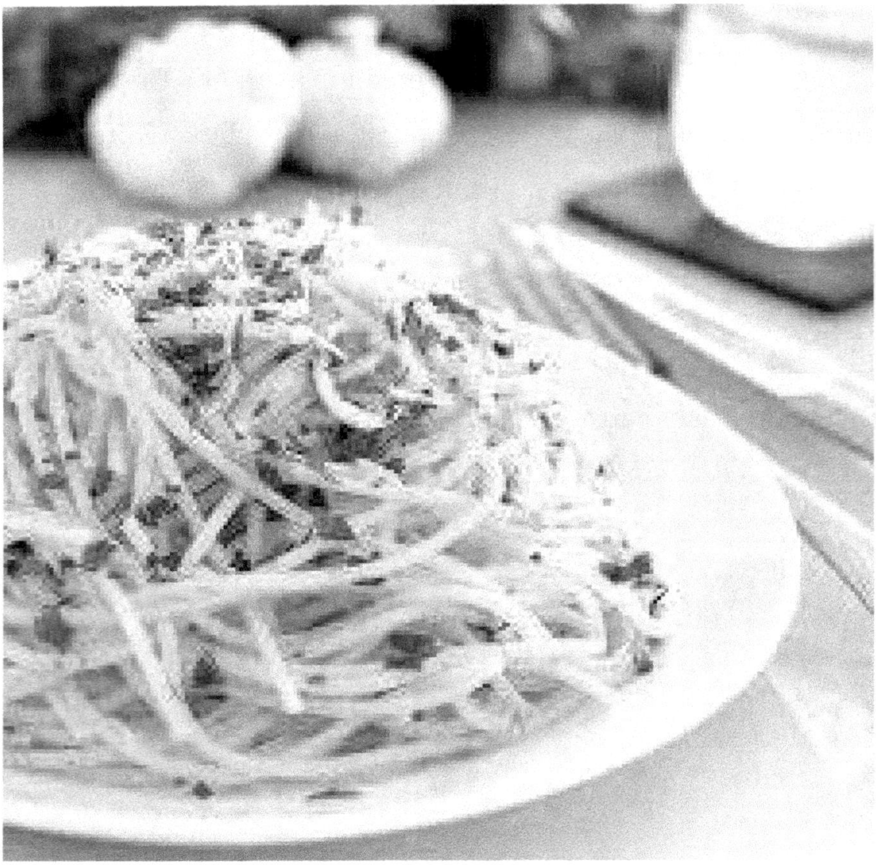

# *Tagliarini Soufflé*

## *Soufflé di Tagliarini*

**Makes 6 servings**

*Some recipes reach my kitchen in a roundabout way. My friend Arthur Schwartz shared this unusual one with me. He learned it from his cooking school partner, Baronessa Cecilia Bellelli Baratta, who in turn learned it from her mother, Elvira. The Baratta family lives in Battipaglia, in the province of Salerno, where Cecilia's father was in the tomato packing business. But for the duration of World War II, the family lived in Parma, where it was much safer.*

*Elvira (at age 91) still cooks many dishes from Parma and claims to have created the idea of a pasta soufflé while living in that region, though in fact other versions do exist. Cecilia points out that northern Italians hardly have a monopoly on egg pasta and cream sauces, no matter what the rest of us think.*

*What is different about this recipe is that it is made with dried egg pasta rather than fresh. Look for* tagliarini, cappellini, *or* cappelli di angelo, *though ordinary thin egg noodles would work as well. The lemon flavor makes the dish seem even lighter than it is.*

## Béchamel Sauce

4 tablespoons unsalted butter

4 tablespoons all-purpose flour

2 cups milk

¾ cup grated Parmigiano-Reggiano

⅛ teaspoon freshly grated nutmeg

1½ teaspoons salt

½ teaspoon freshly ground black pepper

Finely grated zest of 1 lemon

Juice of 1 lemon

4 large eggs, separated

Salt

8 ounces dried tagliarini, or another fine dried egg pasta, broken into 3-inch lengths

4 tablespoons unsalted butter

1 egg white

¼ cup plus 2 tablespoons plain dry bread crumbs

**1.** Prepare the sauce: Melt the butter in a small saucepan over medium heat. Stir in the flour using a whisk and let cook for 2 minutes.

**2.** Whisking constantly, add the milk. Bring to a simmer, stirring frequently. Remove from the heat and stir in the cheese. Allow to cool slightly before stirring in the nutmeg, salt, pepper, lemon zest, and juice.

**3.** Scrape the mixture into a large mixing bowl and let cool to room temperature. (Or, if you are in a hurry, cool the mixture by placing the bowl in another bowl filled with ice water.) Stir in the egg yolks, mixing thoroughly.

**4.** Bring about 3 quarts of water to a boil. Add 2 tablespoons of salt, then the pasta. Boil it until it is only half done. The pasta will be flexible but still hard in the center. Drain well. Transfer the pasta back to the pot it was cooked in and toss with 2 tablespoons of the remaining butter. Let the pasta cool slightly.

**5.** Place a rack in the center of the oven. Preheat the oven to 375°F. Using 1 tablespoon of the remaining butter, grease a 9 × 9 × 2-

inch baking dish. Sprinkle with about $^1/_4$ cup of the bread crumbs, coating the dish well.

**6.** In a large bowl with an electric mixer on medium speed, beat the egg whites with a pinch of salt until soft peaks form. Gently fold the whites into the béchamel sauce. With a rubber spatula, fold the sauce into the pasta a little at a time. Work carefully so as not to deflate the whites too much. Scrape the mixture into the prepared baking dish.

**7.** Sprinkle with the remaining 2 tablespoons bread crumbs. Dot with the remaining 1 tablespoon of butter.

**8.** Bake for 30 minutes or until the soufflé is puffed and lightly golden.

**9.** For maximum lightness, cut into squares and serve immediately. The soufflé will sink slightly as it cools.

# *Spaghetti, Charcoal Burner's Style*

## *Spaghetti alla Carbonara*

**Makes 6 to 8 servings**

*Romans credit the hard-working charcoal delivery man as the inspiration for this quickly made pasta. They say the generous grinding of black pepper resembles specks of coal dust!*

*Some cooks in the United States add cream to the sauce, but this is the way it is made in Rome.*

4 ounces pancetta, cut into thick slices

1 tablespoon olive oil

3 large eggs

Salt and freshly ground black pepper

1 pound spaghetti or linguine

¾ cup freshly grated Pecorino Romano or Parmigiano-Reggiano

**1.** Cut the pancetta into ¼-inch pieces. Pour the oil into a skillet large enough to hold all of the cooked pasta. Add the pancetta.

Cook over medium heat, until the pancetta is golden around the edges, about 10 minutes. Turn off the heat.

**2.** In a medium bowl, beat the eggs with a generous amount of salt and pepper.

**3.** Bring at least 4 quarts of water to a boil in a large pot. Add 2 tablespoons of salt, then the pasta, gently pushing it down until the pasta is completely covered with water. Stir well. Cook over high heat, stirring frequently, until the pasta is al dente, tender yet still firm to the bite. Drain the pasta, reserving some of the cooking water.

**4.** Place the cooked pasta in the pan with the pancetta and toss well over medium heat. Add the eggs and a little of the cooking water. Toss gently until the pasta looks creamy. Sprinkle with cheese and more pepper. Toss well and serve immediately.

# *Bucatini with Tomatoes, Pancetta, and Hot Pepper*

## *Bucatini all'Amatriciana*

**Makes 4 to 6 servings**

*Amatrice is the name of a town in the Abruzzo region. Many people from that area settled in Rome, and this recipe became one of the city's signature dishes. As with all traditions, everyone argues about the right way to uphold it. I once listened to a Roman call-in radio program on the subject that went on for an hour discussing the pros and cons of adding onion.*

*I have tried numerous versions, and this is the way I like it best.* Bucatini, *a very thick spaghetti shape with a hole in the center, is traditional but hard to eat. Unlike spaghetti, linguine, and other long pasta strands, it does not twirl neatly around the fork, especially if it is cooked firm the way the Romans like it. A short thin pasta tube like penne is also good and a lot neater to eat.*

2 tablespoons olive oil

2 ounces sliced pancetta, about 1⁄8 inch thick, chopped into tiny bits

1 medium onion, finely chopped

Pinch of crushed red pepper

½ cup dry white wine

1 (28-ounce) can imported Italian peeled tomatoes, drained and chopped

Salt

1 pound bucatini, perciatelli, or penne

½ cup freshly grated Pecorino Romano

**1.** Pour the oil into a skillet large enough to hold all of the cooked pasta. Add the pancetta, onion, and crushed red pepper. Cook, stirring occasionally, over medium heat, until the pancetta and onion are golden, about 12 minutes.

**2.** Add the wine and bring to a simmer.

**3.** Stir in the tomatoes and salt to taste. Bring the sauce to a simmer and cook, stirring occasionally, until the sauce is thickened, about 25 minutes.

**4.** Bring at least 4 quarts of water to a boil in a large pot. Add 2 tablespoons of salt, then the pasta. Stir well. Cook over high heat, stirring frequently, until the pasta is al dente, tender yet still firm to the bite. Set aside some of the cooking water. Drain the pasta.

**5.** Pour the pasta into the pan with the sauce. Toss the pasta and sauce together over high heat about 1 minute, or until the pasta is coated. Add a little cooking water if the pasta seems dry. Remove from the heat. Add the cheese and toss well. Serve immediately.

## *Penne with Pancetta, Pecorino, and Black Pepper*

### *Penne alla Gricia*

**Makes 4 to 6 servings**

*I was reminded of how good this pasta can be at New York's San Domenico Restaurant, where it was prepared for a luncheon celebrating the cooking of Rome. I had to include it in this collection.*

*Penne alla Gricia is a close relative, and quite possibly the forerunner, of the Bucatini all'Amatriciana at left. Traditional recipes for both have the same ingredients—salted meat, lard, and grated sheep's cheese, which were the typical flavorings for pasta before tomatoes arrived from the New World and were accepted in Italy. Pork lard adds a very good flavor, but olive oil can be substituted if you prefer.*

*In Rome, this is made with* guanciale, *cured pork cheek. Unless you live near an Italian specialty butcher, guanciale is hard to find, but pancetta is very similar. Have the slices cut about ⅛-inch thick, if you can. To make the slices easier to chop, try freezing them briefly on a piece of wax paper.*

2 tablespoons pork lard or olive oil

4 ounces sliced guanciale or pancetta, about ⅛ inch thick, chopped into tiny bits

Salt

1 pound spaghetti

½ cup freshly grated Pecorino Romano

½ teaspoon freshly ground black pepper or more to taste

**1.** In a skillet large enough to hold all of the cooked pasta, heat the lard or olive oil over medium heat. Add the guanciale or pancetta, and cook, stirring frequently, 10 minutes or until crisp and golden brown.

**2.** Bring at least 4 quarts of water to a boil in a large pot. Add 2 tablespoons of salt, then the pasta. Stir well. Cook over high heat, stirring frequently, until the pasta is al dente, tender yet still firm to the bite. Set aside some of the cooking water. Drain the pasta.

**3.** Pour the pasta into the skillet and toss it with the cheese, pepper, and a couple of tablespoons of the water until the pasta is well coated. Serve immediately with more pepper, if desired.

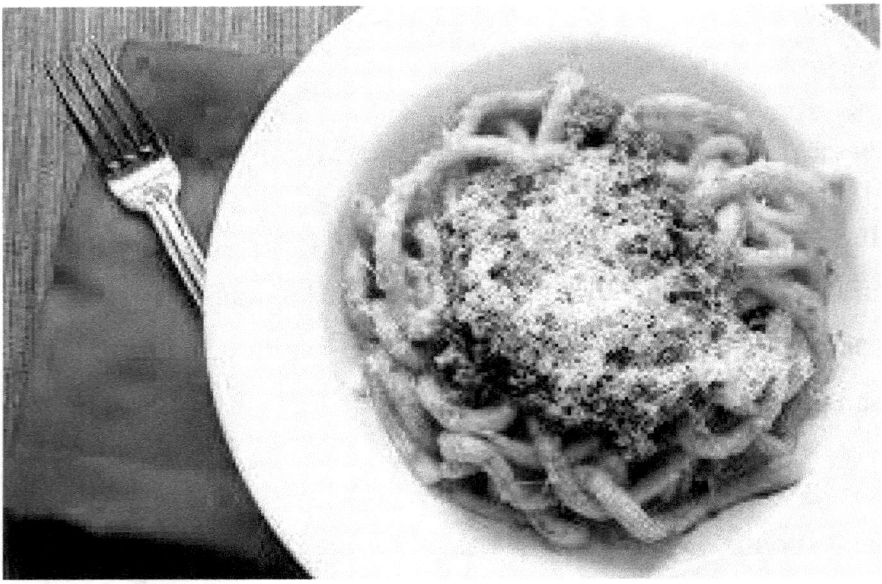

# *Penne with Pork and Cauliflower*

## *Pasta Incaciata*

**Makes 4 to 6 servings**

*My friend Carmella Ragusa showed me how to make this recipe, which she learned when visiting her family in Sicily.*

2 tablespoons olive oil

2 garlic cloves, finely chopped

8 ounces ground pork

1 teaspoon fennel seeds

½ cup dry red wine

1 pound fresh plum tomatoes, peeled, seeded, and chopped, or 2 cups canned imported Italian tomatoes, drained and chopped

Salt and freshly ground black pepper

3 cups cauliflower florets

1 pound penne

About 1 cup freshly grated Pecorino Romano

**1.** Pour the oil into a large skillet. Add the the garlic and cook over medium heat until golden, about 2 minutes. Add the pork and fennel seeds and stir well. Cook, stirring occasionally, until the meat is browned, about 15 minutes.

**2.** Add the wine and simmer 3 minutes, or until most of the liquid evaporates.

**3.** Add the tomatoes and salt and pepper to taste. Simmer 15 minutes or until the sauce is slightly reduced.

**4.** Bring at least 4 quarts of water to a boil in a large pot. Add the cauliflower and 2 tablespoons of salt. Cook until the cauliflower is tender, about 10 minutes. With a slotted spoon, scoop out the cauliflower and drain well. Do not discard the water.

**5.** Add the cauliflower to the sauce and cook, stirring frequently and breaking up the pieces with a spoon, until the sauce is thick, about 10 minutes more.

**6.** Bring the water back to a boil and add the pasta. Cook, stirring frequently, until the pasta is al dente, tender yet still firm to the bite. Set aside some of the cooking water. Drain the pasta.

**7.** Transfer the pasta to a heated serving bowl. Toss the pasta with the sauce, thinning it if necessary with the cooking water. Add the cheese and toss well. Serve immediately.

# *Spaghetti with Vodka Sauce*

## *Spaghetti alla Vodka*

**Makes 4 to 6 servings**

*According to my friend Arthur Schwartz, a cookbook author and food authority, this pasta was invented in the 1970s in Italy as part of an advertising campaign for a major vodka company. I first had it in Rome, but it seems to be more popular now in the United States than it is in Italy.*

¹⁄₄ cup unsalted butter

¹⁄₄ cup finely chopped shallots

2 ounces sliced imported Italian prosciutto, cut into thin strips

1 (28-ounce) can imported Italian peeled tomatoes, drained and coarsely chopped

¹⁄₂ teaspoon crushed red pepper

Salt

¹⁄₂ cup heavy cream

¹⁄₄ cup vodka

1 pound spaghetti or linguine

½ cup freshly grated Parmigiano-Reggiano

**1.** In a skillet large enough to hold all of the cooked pasta, melt the butter over medium heat. Add the shallots and cook until golden, about 2 minutes. Stir in the prosciutto and cook 1 minute.

**2.** Add the tomatoes, crushed red pepper, and salt to taste. Simmer 5 minutes. Stir in the cream and cook, stirring well, for 1 minute more. Add the vodka and cook 2 minutes.

**3.** Bring 4 quarts of water to a boil in a large pot. Add 2 tablespoons of salt, then the pasta, gently pushing it down until the pasta is completely covered with water. Cook over high heat, stirring frequently, until al dente, tender yet still firm to the bite. Set aside some of the cooking water. Drain the pasta.

**4.** Add the pasta to the skillet with the sauce. Toss the pasta in the sauce over high heat until it is well coated. Add a little cooking water if the sauce seems too thick. Stir in the cheese and toss again. Serve immediately.

## *Bow Ties with Asparagus, Cream, and Prosciutto*

### *Farfalle con Asparagi*

**Makes 6 to 8 servings**

*This combination is perfect for a spring menu. I find the cream makes it very rich, so I tend to serve this pasta in small portions as a first course before something simple like grilled veal or chicken. I have added chopped roasted peppers to this pasta and like the combination very much.*

1 pound fresh asparagus, trimmed

Salt

1 cup heavy cream

1 pound farfalle

½ cup freshly grated Parmigiano-Reggiano

2 ounces sliced imported Italian prosciutto, cut crosswise into thin strips

**1.** In a large skillet, bring about 2 inches of water to a boil. Add the asparagus and salt to taste. Cook until the asparagus are just tender and bend slightly when lifted from the water. The cooking time will depend on the thickness of the asparagus. Pat the asparagus dry. Cut them into bite-size pieces.

**2.** Bring the cream to a simmer in a small saucepan. Cook 5 minutes or until slightly thickened.

**3.** Bring a large pot of water to a boil. Add 2 tablespoons of salt, then the pasta. Stir well. Cook over high heat, stirring frequently, until the pasta is al dente, tender yet still firm to the bite. Set aside some of the cooking water. Drain the pasta.

**4.** Pour the pasta, cream, and cheese into a large serving bowl and toss well. Add a little cooking water if the sauce seems too thick. Add the asparagus and prosciutto and toss again. Serve immediately.

# *"Dragged" Penne with Meat Sauce*

## *Penne Strascinate*

**Makes 6 servings**

*I first had this pasta at a little country restaurant in Tuscany, a region in which every cook has her or his own way of making it. It is called "dragged" penne because the pasta finishes cooking as it is stirred in the sauce. This infuses the pasta with the flavor of the sauce.*

¼ cup olive oil

1 medium onion, finely chopped

1 medium carrot, finely chopped

1 tender celery rib, finely chopped

1 garlic clove, very finely chopped

2 tablespoons chopped fresh basil

12 ounces ground veal

½ cup dry red wine

2 cups peeled, seeded, and chopped fresh tomatoes or canned imported Italian peeled tomatoes, drained and chopped

1 cup homemade Meat Broth or Chicken Broth or store-bought beef or chicken broth

Salt and freshly ground black pepper

1 pound penne

½ cup freshly grated Pecorino Romano

½ cup freshly grated Parmigiano-Reggiano

**1.** Pour the oil into a skillet large enough to hold all of the cooked pasta. Add the onion, carrot, celery, garlic, and basil. Cook over medium heat until the vegetables are tender, about 10 minutes.

**2.** Add the veal and cook, stirring frequently to break up any lumps, about 10 minutes. Add the wine and bring to a simmer. Cook 1 minute.

**3.** Stir in the tomatoes, the broth, and salt and pepper to taste. Simmer on low heat 45 minutes, stirring occasionally.

**4.** Bring 4 quarts of water to a boil in a large pot. Add 2 tablespoons of salt, then the pasta. Stir well. Cook over high heat, stirring frequently, until the pasta is almost tender but slightly underdone. Set aside some cooking water. Drain the pasta.

**5.** Add the pasta to the skillet and raise the heat to medium. Cook, stirring the pasta well, for 2 minutes, adding some of the water if necessary. Stir in the cheeses and serve immediately.

# *Spaghetti, Caruso Style*

## *Spaghetti Enrico Caruso*

**Makes 6 servings**

*Enrico Caruso, the great Neapolitan tenor, loved to cook and eat. Pasta was his specialty, and this is said to have been one of his favorites.*

¼ cup olive oil

¼ cup finely chopped shallots or onions

8 ounces chicken livers, trimmed and cut into bite-size pieces

1 teaspoon finely chopped rosemary

Salt and freshly ground black pepper

2 cups peeled, seeded, and chopped fresh tomatoes, or canned imported Italian peeled tomatoes, drained and chopped

1 pound spaghetti or linguine

2 tablespoons unsalted butter

½ cup freshly grated Parmigiano-Reggiano

1. Pour the oil into a skillet large enough to hold all of the pasta. Add the shallots. Cook over medium heat until tender, about 3 minutes. Add the livers, rosemary, and salt and pepper to taste. Cook 2 minutes or until the livers are no longer pink.

2. Stir in the tomatoes and bring to a simmer. Cook 20 minutes or until slightly thickened.

3. Bring 4 quarts of water to a boil in a large pot. Add 2 tablespoons of salt, then the pasta, gently pushing it down until the pasta is completely covered with water. Stir well. Cook over high heat, stirring frequently, until the pasta is al dente, tender yet still firm to the bite. Set aside some of the cooking water. Drain the pasta.

4. Add the spaghetti to the sauce and toss together 1 minute over high heat. Add a little cooking water if the sauce seems too thick. Add the butter and cheese and toss again. Serve immediately.

# *Penne with Beans and Pancetta*

## *Penne e Fagioli*

**Makes 4 to 6 servings**

*Some pasta and bean recipes are thick and souplike, with equal parts beans and pasta. This Tuscan version is really pasta with a bean and tomato sauce.*

2 tablespoons olive oil

2½ ounces pancetta, finely chopped

1 medium onion, finely chopped

1 large garlic clove, peeled and finely chopped

2 cups drained cooked or canned cranberry or cannellini beans

1½ pounds plum tomatoes, peeled, seeded, and chopped, or 3 cups canned imported Italian tomatoes, drained and chopped

Salt to taste

1 pound penne

Freshly ground black pepper

½ cup chopped flat-leaf parsley

½ cup freshly grated Parmigiano-Reggiano

**1.** Pour the oil into a large saucepan. Add the pancetta. Cook over medium heat, stirring occasionally, 10 minutes or until lightly browned. Add the onion and cook until it is tender and golden, about 10 minutes.

**2.** Stir in the garlic and cook 1 minute more. Add the beans, tomatoes, and salt and pepper. Cook 5 minutes.

**3.** Bring about 4 quarts of water to a boil in a large pot. Add 2 tablespoons of salt, then the pasta. Stir well. Cook over high heat, stirring frequently, until the pasta is al dente, tender yet still firm to the bite. Set aside some of the cooking water. Drain the pasta.

**4.** In a large warm serving bowl, toss the pasta with the sauce and parsley. Add a little of the cooking water, if needed. Add the cheese and toss again. Serve with freshly grated Parmigiano-Reggiano.

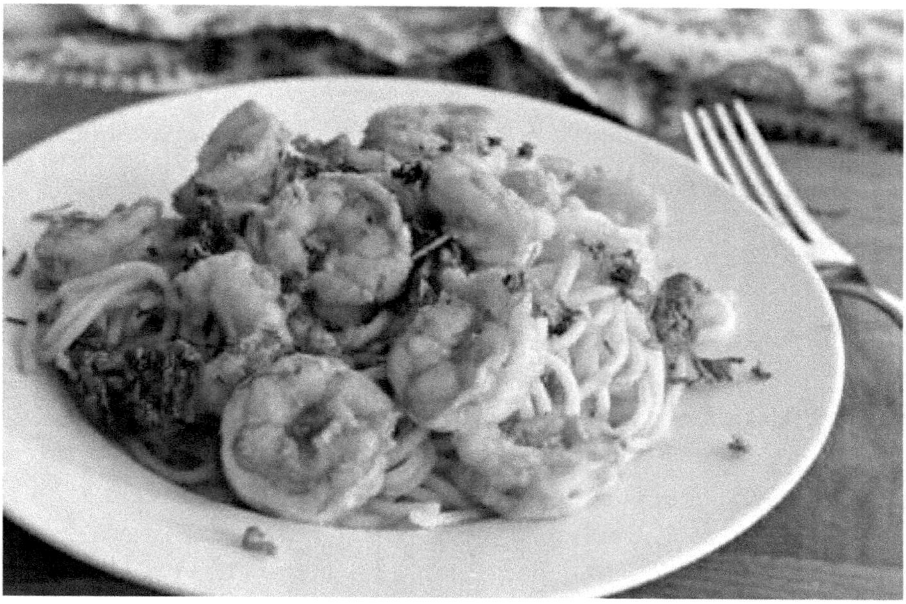

# *Pasta with Chickpeas*

## *Pasta e Ceci*

**Makes 4 servings**

*A drizzle of extra-virgin olive oil is the perfect finishing touch for pasta with chickpeas. If you want to make it spicy, try it with some of the Holy Oil.*

2 tablespoons olive oil

2 ounces thick-sliced pancetta, finely chopped

1 medium onion, chopped

1 pound tomatoes, peeled, seeded, and chopped

1 tablespoon chopped fresh sage

Pinch of crushed red pepper

Salt

2 cups drained cooked or canned chickpeas

8 ounces small pasta, such as elbow or ditali

Extra-virgin olive oil

1. Pour the oil into a large saucepan. Add the pancetta and onion and cook, stirring occasionally, over medium heat, about 10 minutes or until tender and golden.

2. Add the tomatoes, 1/2 cup water, sage, red pepper, and salt to taste. Bring to a simmer and cook 15 minutes. Add the chickpeas and cook 10 minutes more.

3. Bring about 4 quarts of water to a boil in a large pot. Stir in 2 tablespoons of salt, then the pasta. Stir well. Cook, stirring frequently, until the pasta is tender yet firm to the bite. Set aside some of the cooking water. Drain the pasta.

4. Add the pasta to the pan with the sauce. Stir well and bring to a simmer, adding some of the cooking water if needed. Serve immediately.

# *Rigatoni Rigoletto*

## *Pasta al Rigoletto*

**Makes 6 servings**

*This pasta is named for Rigoletto, the tragic hero of Verdi's glorious opera. The story is set in Mantua, where this pasta is well known.*

2 or 3 Italian-style pork sausages (about 12 ounces)

2 tablespoons olive oil

1 medium onion, finely chopped

2 garlic cloves, finely chopped

4 tablespoons tomato paste

2 cups water

2 cups cooked dried cranberry or cannellini beans, lightly drained

Salt and freshly ground black pepper

1 pound rigatoni

1 tablespoon unsalted butter

¼ cup finely chopped fresh basil

½ cup freshly grated Parmigiano-Reggiano

**1.** Remove the casings from the sausages and finely chop the meat.

**2.** Pour the oil into a saucepan large enough to hold all of the ingredients. Add the onion, sausage meat, and garlic. Cook over medium heat, stirring frequently, until the onions are tender and the sausage is lightly browned, about 15 minutes.

**3.** Add the tomato paste and water. Bring to a simmer and cook 20 minutes or until slightly thickened.

**4.** Add the beans and salt and pepper to taste. Cook 10 minutes, mashing some of the beans with the back of a spoon to make the sauce creamy.

**5.** Bring at least 4 quarts of water to a boil in a large pot. Add 2 tablespoons of salt, then the pasta. Stir well. Cook over high heat, stirring frequently, until the pasta is al dente, tender yet still firm to the bite. Set aside some of the cooking water. Drain the pasta.

**6.** Add the pasta to the pan with the sauce, toss together, and cook 1 minute, adding a little of the water if needed. Stir in the butter and basil. Add the cheese and toss again. Serve immediately.

# *Anna's Fried Spaghetti*

## *Spaghetti Fritti alla Anna*

**Makes 4 servings**

*When my husband and I and a group of friends visited cooking school owner and teacher Anna Tasca Lanza at her family's farm and wine estate at Regaleali, Sicily, we shared numerous meals. Toward the end of our stay, we decided to make a casual lunch with whatever was in the refrigerator. While the rest of us were busy slicing bread and cheese, pouring wine, and making a salad, Anna took out some leftover spaghetti and poured it into a heavy skillet. In a few minutes, the pasta had turned into a crunchy golden cake that everyone devoured. Anna seemed surprised that we had enjoyed it so much and said it was just something that you can do with leftover pasta. My friend Judith Weber eventually got more information about how she had made it and passed the recipe along to me. This is great for a midnight supper, and it can be made with just about any type of leftover pasta, though long strands are best because they will stick together.*

4 to 8 ounces cold leftover spaghetti with Sicilian Tomato Sauce or Marinara Sauce

3 tablespoons olive oil

2 tablespoons grated Pecorino Romano

**1.** Prepare the spaghetti with tomato sauce if necessary. Chill at least 1 hour or overnight.

**2.** In a large nonstick skillet, heat 2 tablespoons of the oil over medium heat. Sprinkle the oil with 1 tablespoon of the cheese and immediately add the pasta to the pan, pressing it flat with the back of a spoon. The pasta should be no more than $^3/_4$ inch deep.

**3.** Cook the pasta, flattening it occasionally against the pan, until golden brown and crisp on the bottom, about 20 minutes. Slide a thin spatula underneath the pasta occasionally to make sure that it is not sticking.

**4.** When the pasta is nicely browned, remove the skillet from heat. Slide a spatula under the pasta to be sure that the it is not stuck. Place a large inverted plate on top of the skillet. Protecting your hands with oven mitts, invert the skillet and plate so that the pasta cake falls out of the skillet onto the plate.

**5.** Add the remaining oil and cheese to the skillet. Slide the pasta cake with the crisp side up back into the pan. Cook the same way as the first side until browned and crisp, about 15 minutes more. Cut into wedges and serve hot.

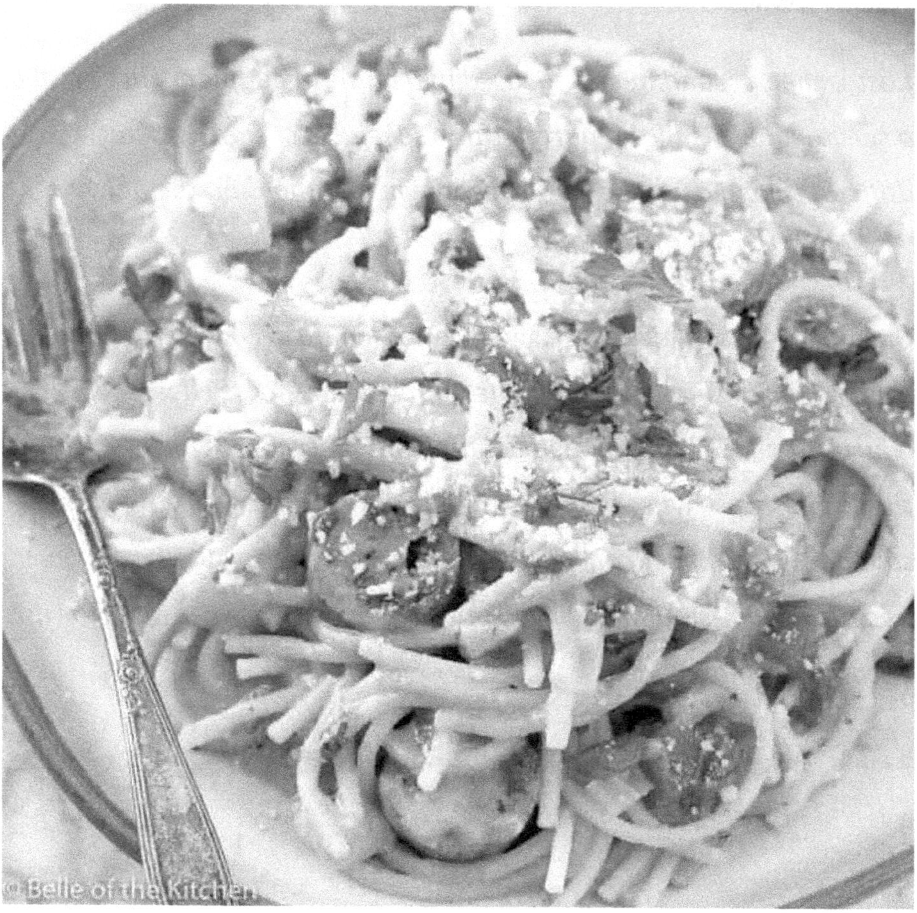

# *Eggplant Pasta Timbale*

## *Pasta al Timballo*

**Makes 6 servings**

*Pasta, cheeses, and meats encased in a dome of eggplant slices make a spectacular dish for a party or any special occasion. It is not difficult to make, but be very careful when unmolding the heavy timbale hot from the oven.*

*In Sicily, this is made with* caciocavallo, *semifirm cow's milk cheese sold in a pear-shaped casing. The name means horse cheese, and why it is called that has been debated for centuries. Some historians think the cheese was originally made with mare's milk, while others say that it was once transported on horseback suspended from poles. Caciocavallo is similar to provolone, which can be substituted, or use Pecorino Romano.*

2 medium eggplants (about 1 pound each)

Salt

Olive oil

1 medium onion, chopped

1 garlic clove, finely chopped

8 ounces ground beef

8 ounces Italian pork sausages, skinned and chopped

2 pounds fresh tomatoes, peeled, seeded, and chopped, or 1 (28-ounce) can imported Italian peeled tomatoes, chopped

1 cup fresh or frozen peas

Freshly ground black pepper

1 pound perciatelli or bucatini

12 ounces mozzarella, chopped

1 cup freshly grated caciocavallo or Pecorino Romano

3 ounces salami, chopped

2 tablespoons chopped fresh basil

2 hard cooked eggs, sliced

**1.** Cut the eggplant lengthwise into 1/4-inch thick slices. Sprinkle the slices generously with salt and place them in a colander to drain at least 30 minutes. Rinse the slices and blot dry.

2. Heat 1/4-inch of oil in a large skillet over medium heat. Fry the slices a few at a time until lightly browned on both sides, about 5 minutes per side. Drain on paper towels.

3. Pour the oil into a large saucepan. Add the onion and garlic and cook over medium heat, stirring frequently, until the onion is softened, about 5 minutes. Add the beef and sausage meat. Cook, stirring often, until lightly browned, about 10 minutes.

4. Add the tomatoes and salt and pepper to taste. Cook on low heat 20 minutes. Add the peas and cook 10 minutes more or until the sauce is thickened.

5. Bring at least 4 quarts of water to a boil in a large pot. Add 2 tablespoons of salt, then the pasta. Stir well. Cook over high heat, stirring frequently, until the pasta is tender but still very firm. Drain the pasta and return it to the pot. Toss the pasta with the sauce. Let cool 5 minutes.

6. Line a 4-quart ovenproof bowl or baking dish with foil, pressing it smoothly against the sides. Brush the foil with olive oil. Starting in the center of the bowl, arrange half the eggplant slices, overlapping slightly against the inside and reserving a few slices for the top.

7. Add the mozzarella, grated cheese, salami, and basil to the pan with the pasta and toss well. Add half the pasta to the prepared bowl, being careful not to disturb the eggplant. Arrange the egg slices over the pasta. Top with the remaining pasta and the reserved eggplant slices. Press down lightly.

8. Place a rack in the center of the oven. Preheat the oven to 400°F. Bake 45 to 60 minutes, or until hot in the center, 140°F measured on an instant-read thermometer. (Exact baking time will depend on the diameter of the bowl.)

9. Let the timbale stand 15 minutes. Invert the bowl onto a serving plate. Remove the bowl and gently peel off the foil. Serve immediately.

# *Baked Ziti*

## *Ziti al Forno*

**Makes 8 to 12 servings**

*Baked pasta dishes like this one are popular all over southern Italy. At a time when few homes had ovens, the pans of pasta would be brought to the local bakery to be cooked after the baker had finished making the day's bread.*

4 cups Neapolitan Ragù

Salt

1 pound ziti, penne, or rigatoni

1 pound whole or part-skim ricotta

1 cup freshly grated Pecorino Romano or Parmigiano-Reggiano cheese

12 ounces fresh mozzarella, chopped or shredded

**1.** Prepare the ragù, if necessary. Then, bring 4 quarts of water to a boil in a large pot. Add 2 tablespoons of salt, then the pasta. Stir well. Cook over high heat, stirring frequently, until almost tender. Drain the pasta.

2. In a large bowl, toss the pasta with 2 cups of the ragù, 1 cup of the ricotta, and half the grated cheese. Slice some of the meatballs and sausages from the ragù and stir them into the pasta. (The remaining meats can be served as a second course.)

3. Place a rack in the center of the oven. Preheat the oven to 350°F. Spread half the ziti in a 13 × 9 × 2–inch baking dish. Spread the remaining ricotta on top. Sprinkle with the mozzarella. Pour on 1 cup of the sauce. Top with the remaining ziti and another cup of sauce. Sprinkle with the remaining 1/2 cup grated cheese. Cover the dish securely with foil.

4. Bake the ziti 45 minutes. Uncover and bake 15 to 30 minutes more, or until the blade of a thin knife inserted into the center feels hot and the sauce is bubbling around the edges. Cool 15 minutes on a wire rack. Serve hot.

# *Sicilian Baked Pasta*

## *Pasta al Forno alla Siciliana*

**Makes 12 servings**

*My husband's Sicilian family looked forward to eating this pasta on special occasions like Christmas and Easter. It was a specialty of his grandmother, Adele Amico, who came from Palermo.*

Anellini, *"little rings," are the typical pasta shape used, but they can be hard to find.* Fusilli lunghi, "*long fusilli," or* bucatini, *thick spaghetti with a hole in the center, are good substitutes. This is a perfect party dish, as it can be made in stages or completely assembled a day ahead of time, and it serves a crowd.*

*If you don't feel comfortable unmolding the pasta, it can be cut into squares and served directly from the pan. A 20- to 30-minute rest after baking helps the pasta to hold its shape.*

### Sauce

¼ cup olive oil

1 medium onion, finely chopped

2 garlic cloves, finely chopped

¼ cup tomato paste

4 (28-ounce) cans imported Italian peeled tomatoes

Salt and freshly ground black pepper

¼ cup chopped fresh basil

## Filling

2 tablespoons olive oil

½ pound ground beef

½ pound ground pork

1 garlic clove, very finely chopped

Salt and freshly ground black pepper

1 cup fresh or frozen peas

2 tablespoons unsalted butter, softened

1 cup plain dry bread crumbs

2 pounds anellini or perciatelli

Salt

½ cup freshly grated Parmigiano-Reggiano

½ cup freshly grated Pecorino Romano

1 cup imported provolone, diced

**1.** Prepare the sauce: Pour the oil into a large saucepan. Add the onion and garlic. Cook over medium heat 10 minutes or until the onion and garlic are tender and golden. Stir in the tomato paste and cook 2 minutes.

**2.** Add the tomatoes and bring to a simmer. Add salt and pepper to taste and cook 1 hour or until the sauce is thickened, stirring occasionally. Stir in the basil.

**3.** Prepare the filling: Heat the oil in a large skillet over medium heat. Add the meats, garlic, and salt and pepper to taste. Cook 10 minutes, stirring to break up the lumps. When the meat is browned, add two cups of the prepared tomato sauce. Bring to a simmer and cook until thickened, about 20 minutes. Stir in the peas. Let cool slightly.

**4.** Smear the butter over the bottom and sides of a 13 × 9 × 2-inch baking pan. Coat the pan with the bread crumbs, patting them so that they adhere.

**5.** Place a rack in the center of the oven. Preheat the oven to 375°F. Bring at least 4 quarts of water to a boil in each of two large pots. Add 3 tablespoons of salt to each pot, then the pasta. Stir well. Cook over high heat, stirring frequently, until the pasta is tender but slightly underdone. Drain the pasta and return it to the pot. Toss the pasta with 3 cups of the plain tomato sauce and the grated cheeses.

**6.** Carefully spoon half the pasta into the prepared pan, trying not to disturb the bread crumbs. Spoon the meat filling evenly over the pasta. Scatter the cheese cubes on top. Spoon the remaining pasta over all. Flatten the contents of the pan with a spoon.

**7.** Have ready a cooling rack and a large tray or cutting board the size of the pan. Bake 60 to 90 minutes or until the pasta is heated through and crusty on top. Let the pasta cool in the pan on the rack 30 minutes. Slide a small knife around the edges of the pan. Protecting your hands with oven mitts, invert the pasta onto the tray or cutting board. Cut into squares and serve warm with the remaining tomato sauce.

# *Sophia Loren's Baked Pasta*

## *Pasta al Forno alla Loren*

**Makes 8 to 10 servings**

*The actress Sophia Loren loves to cook and has even written cookbooks. Her real last name is Scicolone, the same as mine, though my name comes from my husband and his Sicilian family. Sophia is from Naples, like my grandparents, though my maiden name was Scotto. I am often asked if we are related. We are not, though I do admire Sophia's beauty and talent, both as an actress and a cook.*

*This is my interpretation of a baked pasta recipe I once heard her describe as a favorite dish for company. If you have prepared the dish ahead and stored it in the refrigerator, be sure to add at least a half hour to the baking time.*

4 cups Bologna-Style Sauce or other meat and tomato sauce

4 cups Béchamel Sauce

Salt

1½ pounds penne, ziti, or mostaccioli

1 cup freshly grated Parmigiano-Reggiano

1. Prepare the two sauces, if necessary. Then, butter a 13 × 9 × 2-inch baking pan.

2. Bring at least 4 quarts of water to a boil in a large pot. Add 2 tablespoons of salt, then the pasta. Stir well. Cook over high heat, stirring frequently, until the pasta is almost tender. Drain the pasta.

3. Place a rack in the center of the oven. Preheat the oven to 400°F. Set aside 1/4 cup of the cheese. Toss the pasta with half of the Bolognese sauce. Spread about 1/3 of the pasta in the pan. Spoon on about 1/3 of the Béchamel sauce and cheese. Dot with additional Bolognese sauce.

4. Repeat, adding two more layers, using all of the ingredients. Sprinkle with the reserved cheese.

5. Cover the pan with foil. Bake until bubbling around the edges and the blade of a thin knife inserted into the center feels hot, about 45 minutes. Uncover and bake 15 minutes more. Remove the pasta from the oven. Cool 15 minutes on a wire rack. Serve hot.

# *Linguine with Clam Sauce*

## *Linguine alle Vongole*

**Makes 4 to 6 servings**

*Use the smallest clams you can find, such as Manila clams or littlenecks. New Zealand cockles have become widely available in my area and may have in your area, too. These work well also. Italians use dime-size* vongole, *tender, hard-shell clams with beautiful zigzag markings. Either these clams are not very sandy, or they are well cleaned before they are cooked, because Italians do not bother to remove the clams from their shells before making the sauce.*

*Linguine with clam sauce should not be served with grated cheese.*

3 pounds small hard-shell clams or New Zealand cockles, well scrubbed

⅓ cup extra-virgin olive oil, plus more for drizzling

4 garlic cloves, finely chopped

2 tablespoon chopped fresh flat-leaf parsley

Pinch of crushed red pepper

1 pound linguine

Salt

**1.** Place the clams in a large pot with $^1/_4$ cup water over medium-high heat. Cover the pot and cook until the liquid is boiling and the clams begin to open. Remove the opened clams with a slotted spoon and transfer to a bowl. Continue cooking the unopened clams. Discard any that refuse to open. Reserve the clam juices.

**2.** Working over a small bowl to catch the juices, scrape the clams from the shells, placing them in another bowl. Pour all of the liquid from the pot into the bowl with the juices. If the clams are sandy, rinse them one at a time in the clam juices. Pass the liquid through a fine-mesh strainer lined with cheesecloth.

**3.** Pour the oil into a skillet large enough to hold the cooked pasta. Add the garlic, parsley, and crushed red pepper. Cook over medium heat until the garlic is golden, about 2 minutes. Add the clam juices. Cook until the liquid is reduced by half. Stir in the clams. Cook 1 minute more.

**4.** Meanwhile, bring at least 4 quarts of water to a boil in a large pot. Add 2 tablespoons of salt, then the linguine, gently pushing it down until the pasta is completely covered with water. Stir well. Cook, stirring frequently, until the linguine is al dente, tender yet still firm to the bite. Drain the pasta.

**5.** Transfer the pasta to the skillet with the sauce and toss well over high heat. Add a drizzle of extra-virgin olive oil and toss again. Serve immediately.

# *Tuscan Spaghetti with Clams*

## *Spaghetti alla Viareggina*

**Makes 4 to 6 servings**

*Here is another version of spaghetti with clams as it is made in Viareggio, on the coast of Tuscany. Onion, wine, and tomatoes give the sauce a more complex flavor.*

3 pounds small hard-shell clams or New Zealand cockles, well scrubbed

Salt

⅓ cup olive oil

1 small onion, finely chopped

2 garlic cloves, finely chopped

Pinch of crushed red pepper

1½ cups peeled, seeded, and chopped fresh tomatoes or drained and chopped canned imported Italian tomatoes

½ cup dry white wine

2 tablespoons chopped fresh flat-leaf parsley

1 pound spaghetti or linguine

**1.** Place the clams in a large pot with $^{1}/_{4}$ cup water over medium-high heat. Cover the pot and cook until the liquid is boiling and the clams begin to open. Remove the opened clams with a slotted spoon and transfer to a bowl. Continue cooking the unopened clams. Discard any that do not open.

**2.** Working over a small bowl to catch the juices, scrape the clams from the shells, placing them in another bowl. Pour all of the liquid from the pot into the bowl with the juices. If the clams are sandy, rinse them one at a time in the clam juices. Pass the liquid through a fine-mesh strainer lined with cheesecloth.

**3.** Pour the oil into a large saucepan. Add the onion and cook, stirring frequently, over medium heat until the onion is golden, about 10 minutes. Add the garlic and crushed red pepper and cook 2 minutes more.

**4.** Stir in the tomatoes, wine, and strained clam juice. Simmer 20 minutes or until the sauce is reduced and thickened.

**5.** Bring at least 4 quarts of water to a boil in a large pot. Add 2 tablespoons of salt, then the pasta, gently pushing it down until the pasta is completely covered with water. Stir well. Cook over high heat, stirring frequently, until the pasta is al dente, tender yet still firm to the bite. Set aside some of the cooking water. Drain the pasta.

6. Stir the clams and parsley into the sauce. Add some of the water if needed. In a heated serving bowl, toss the sauce and pasta together. Serve immediately.

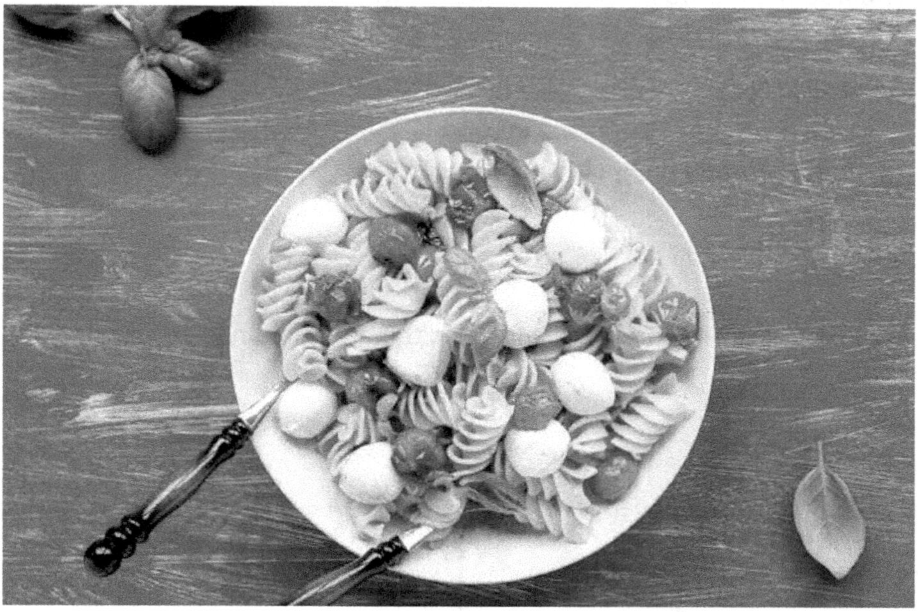

# *Linguine with Anchovies and Spicy Tomato Sauce*

## *Linguine alla Puttanesca*

**Makes 4 to 6 servings**

*The usual explanation for the Italian name for this tasty sauce is that it was invented by either Roman or Neapolitan streetwalkers who had little time for cooking but wanted a hot, tasty meal.*

¼ cup olive oil

3 garlic cloves, very finely chopped

Pinch of crushed red pepper

1 (28-ounce) can imported Italian peeled tomatoes, drained and chopped

Salt

6 anchovy fillets, chopped

½ cup chopped Gaeta or other mild black olives

2 tablespoons chopped rinsed capers

2 tablespoons chopped fresh flat-leaf parsley

1 pound linguine or spaghetti

1. Pour the oil into a skillet large enough to hold all of the cooked pasta. Add the garlic and the crushed red pepper. Cook until the garlic is golden, about 2 minutes.

2. Add the tomatoes and a pinch of salt. Bring to a simmer and cook 15 to 20 minutes or until the sauce is thickened.

3. Add the anchovies, olives, and capers and simmer 2 to 3 minutes more. Stir in the parsley.

4. Bring at least 4 quarts of water to a boil in a large pot. Add the linguine and salt to taste. Gently push the pasta down until it is completely covered with water. Cook, stirring frequently, until the pasta is al dente, tender yet still firm to the bite. Set aside some of the cooking water. Drain the pasta.

5. Add the pasta to the skillet with the sauce. Toss 1 minute over high heat, adding a little of the cooking water if needed. Serve immediately.

# *Linguine with Crab and Little Tomatoes*

## *Linguine al Granchio*

**Makes 4 to 6 servings**

*In Naples, tiny dried chiles add flavor to many seafood sauces, but use any hot red pepper sparingly, as it can overwhelm the delicacy of the crab meat. The same goes for the garlic, which in this recipe is used just to flavor the cooking oil, then removed before the tomatoes and crab are added.*

⅓ cup olive oil

3 large garlic cloves, crushed

Pinch of crushed red pepper

2 pints cherry or grape tomatoes, halved or quartered if large

Salt and freshly ground black pepper

8 ounces fresh lump crabmeat, picked over to remove bits of shell, or chopped cooked lobster

8 fresh basil leaves, torn into bits

1 pound linguine

1. Pour the oil into a large skillet. Add the garlic cloves and red pepper and cook over medium heat, pressing down on the garlic once or twice with the back of a spoon, until the garlic is deep golden, about 4 minutes. Remove the garlic with a slotted spoon.

2. Add the tomatoes and salt and pepper to taste. Cook, stirring frequently, until the tomatoes are softened and have released their juices, about 10 minutes.

3. Gently stir in the crab and basil. Remove from the heat.

4. Bring at least 4 quarts of water to a boil in a large pot. Add 2 tablespoons of salt, then the pasta, gently pushing it down until the pasta is completely covered with water. Stir well. Cook over high heat, stirring frequently, until the linguine is al dente, tender yet still firm to the bite.

5. Drain the pasta, reserving a little of the cooking water. Add the pasta to the pan with the sauce, adding a little of the water if it seems dry. Toss over high heat 1 minute. Serve immediately.

# *Linguine with Mixed Seafood Sauce*

## *Linguine ai Frutti di Mare*

**Makes 4 to 6 servings**

*Sweet little grape tomatoes are full of flavor like the* pomodorini della collina, *little hillside tomatoes, grown around Naples. If grape tomatoes are not available, use cherry tomatoes or chopped fresh plum tomatoes instead.*

*This sauce can be prepared in the brief time it takes to cook the pasta. To be sure that nothing gets overcooked, have all of the ingredients and needed equipment ready before starting. To save time and effort, you can use precut calamari (squid) rings.*

1 pound cleaned calamari (squid)

6 tablespoons extra-virgin olive oil, plus more for drizzling

Salt

1 pound medium shrimp, shelled and deveined

2 large garlic cloves, very finely chopped

¼ cup chopped fresh flat-leaf parsley

Pinch of crushed red pepper

1 pint grape or cherry tomatoes, halved

1 pound small hard-shell clams or mussels, cleaned and shelled as directed in steps 1 and 2 of Linguine with Clam Sauce, including juice

1 pound linguine or thin spaghetti

**1.** Cut the calamari bodies into 1/2-inch rings and the base of the tentacles in half crosswise. Cut the shrimp into 1/2-inch pieces. Pat the seafood dry.

**2.** In a skillet large enough to hold all of the ingredients, heat 4 tablespoons of the oil over medium-high heat. Add the calamari and salt to taste. Cook, stirring often, until the calamari are just opaque, about 2 minutes. Scoop the calamari out with a slotted spoon and transfer to a plate. Add the shrimp and salt, to taste, to the pan. Cook, stirring, until the shrimp are just pink, about 1 minute. Transfer the shrimp to the plate with the calamari.

**3.** Add the remaining 2 tablespoons of the oil, and the garlic, parsley, and red pepper to the pan. Cook, stirring, until the garlic is golden, about 2 minutes. Add the tomatoes and clam juice. Cook 5 minutes or until the tomatoes are tender. Stir in the calamari, shrimp and clams.

**4.** Bring at least 4 quarts of water to a boil in a large pot. Add 2 tablespoons of salt, then the pasta, gently pushing it down until the pasta is completely covered with water. Stir well. Cook over high heat, stirring frequently, until the pasta is al dente, tender yet still firm to the bite. Drain the pasta, reserving some of the cooking water.

**5.** Add the pasta to the pan with the seafood. Cook over high heat, tossing the pasta with the sauce, for 30 seconds. Add a little cooking water if needed. Drizzle with extra-virgin olive oil and toss again. Serve hot.

# *Thin Spaghetti with Bottarga*

## *Spaghettini con Bottarga*

**Makes 4 to 6 servings**

*Bottarga is the dried salted roe of mullet, tuna, or other fish. Most of it comes from Sardinia or Sicily. It is sold in a whole piece in the refrigerator case of many seafood markets and gourmet shops and shaved or grated with a vegetable peeler or cheese grater. There is also a dried, powdered type that is sold in jars. It is convenient, but I prefer the refrigerated variety. The flavor of bottarga is somewhere between that of caviar and top-quality anchovies.*

⅓ cup extra-virgin olive oil

2 garlic cloves, finely chopped

2 tablespoons chopped fresh flat-leaf parsley

Pinch of crushed red pepper

Salt

1 pound thin spaghetti

3 to 4 tablespoons shaved or grated bottarga

**1.** Pour the oil into a skillet large enough to hold all of the pasta. Add the garlic, parsley, and pepper. Cook over medium heat until the garlic is golden, about 2 minutes.

**2.** Bring at least 4 quarts of water to a boil in a large pot. Add 2 tablespoons of salt, then the pasta. Stir well, gently pushing the pasta down until it is completely covered with water. Cook over high heat, stirring frequently, until the pasta is al dente, tender yet still firm to the bite. Drain the pasta, reserving some of the cooking water.

**3.** Add the pasta to the skillet and toss well 1 minute over high heat Add some of the cooking water if needed. Sprinkle with the bottarga and toss again. Serve immediately.

# *Venetian Whole-Wheat Spaghetti in Anchovy Sauce*

## *Bigoli in Salsa*

**Makes 4 to 6 servings**

*In Venice, thick whole-wheat spaghetti is handmade with a special device called a torchio that works something like a meat grinder. The dough is forced through small holes in the torchio and emerges as long strands. For this recipe, which is a Venetian classic, I use dried whole-wheat spaghetti.*

¼ cup olive oil

2 medium red onions, halved and thinly sliced

½ cup dry white wine

1 (3-ounce) jar anchovy fillets

Salt

1 pound whole-wheat spaghetti

Freshly ground black pepper

**1.** Pour the oil into a skillet large enough to hold all of the pasta. Add the onions and cook over medium heat until the onions are golden, about 10 minutes. Add the wine and cook, stirring frequently, until the onions are soft but not browned, about 15 minutes more.

**2.** Drain the anchovies, reserving the oil. Add the anchovies to the skillet and stir. Cook 10 minutes more, stirring often, until the anchovies dissolve.

**3.** Bring at least 4 quarts of water to a boil in a large pot. Add 2 tablespoons of salt, then the pasta. Stir well, gently pushing the pasta down until it is completely covered with water. Cook over high heat, stirring frequently, until the pasta is al dente, tender yet still firm to the bite. Set aside some of the cooking water. Drain the pasta.

**4.** Add the pasta to the pan with the sauce, and toss together 1 minute over high heat, adding a little of the water if needed. Drizzle with some of the reserved anchovy oil if desired, and top with freshly ground pepper. Serve immediately.

# *Capri-Style Spaghetti*

## *Spaghetti alla Caprese*

**Makes 4 to 6 servings**

*Fish and cheese are rarely combined in Italy, because the sharpness of the cheese may overwhelm the delicacy of the fish. But for every rule, there is an exception. Here is a pasta from the island of Capri that combines two types of fish with mozzarella. The flavors work because the cheese is mild and rich, yet easily dominated by the anchovies and tuna.*

⅓ cup olive oil

2 cups peeled, seeded, and chopped fresh tomatoes or drained and chopped canned imported Italian tomatoes

Salt

4 anchovy fillets, chopped

1 (7-ounce) can tuna in olive oil, drained and chopped

12 Gaeta or other mild black olives, pitted and chopped

Freshly ground black pepper

1 pound spaghetti

Salt

4 ounces fresh mozzarella, diced

**1.** In a skillet large enough to hold the cooked pasta, heat the olive oil over medium heat. Add the tomatoes and salt to taste. Cook, stirring occasionally, 10 to 15 minutes or until the tomato juices have evaporated. Turn off the heat.

**2.** Stir the chopped ingredients into the tomato sauce. Add pepper to taste.

**3.** Bring at least 4 quarts of water to a boil in a large pot. Add 2 tablespoons of salt, then the pasta. Stir well, gently pushing the pasta down until it is completely covered with water. Cook over high heat, stirring frequently, until the pasta is al dente, tender yet still firm to the bite. Drain the pasta, reserving some of the cooking water.

**4.** Add the pasta to the pan with the sauce and toss well 1 minute over medium heat. Add a little water if the pasta seems dry. Add the mozzarella and toss again. Serve immediately.

# *Linguine with Shrimp, Venetian Style*

## *Linguine al Gamberi alla Veneta*

**Makes 6 servings**

*Perhaps because their city was once a major trading port with the East, Venetian cooks have always been open to experimentation. This linguine, for example, is flavored with a slice of fresh ginger, which is not often used in Italian cooking but works wonderfully with shrimp.*

1½ pounds large shrimp, shelled and deveined

½ cup olive oil

3 garlic cloves, finely chopped

¼-inch thick piece fresh ginger, peeled

Pinch of crushed red pepper

Salt to taste

1 tablespoon fresh lemon juice

1 cup dry white wine

2 tablespoons chopped fresh flat-leaf parsley

1 pound linguine

**1.** Rinse the shrimp and pat them dry. Cut each shrimp into 1/2-inch pieces.

**2.** Pour the oil into a skillet large enough to hold all of the cooked pasta. Add the garlic, ginger, and crushed red pepper. Cook over medium heat until the garlic is golden, about 2 minutes. Add the shrimp and a big pinch of salt. Cook, stirring, until the shrimp are cooked through, about 2 minutes. Add the lemon juice and wine and bring to a simmer. Cook 2 minutes. Stir in the parsley. Remove from the heat.

**3.** Bring at least 4 quarts of water to a boil in a large pot. Add 2 tablespoons of salt, then the pasta. Stir well, gently pushing the pasta down until it is completely covered with water. Cook over high heat, stirring frequently, until the pasta is al dente, tender yet still firm to the bite. Drain the pasta, reserving some of the cooking water.

**4.** Add the pasta to the skillet and toss over high heat 1 minute until well mixed. Add a little of the cooking water if needed. Remove the ginger. Serve immediately.

## *Pasta with Sardines and Fennel*

### *Pasta con le Sarde*

**Makes 6 servings**

*Sicilians are passionate about this dish, and every cook claims to have the best and most authentic recipe. Some add tomatoes, and some stew the sardines along with the fennel, but I prefer this method of cooking the sardines separately and layering them with the pasta and saving the tomatoes for another recipe.*

*Fennel grows wild all over Sicily, and the green fronds are used to make this pasta. Cultivated fennel does not have the same flavor, but the wild fennel is not widely available here. I use a combination of fresh dill and cultivated fennel to approximate the flavor of this classic Sicilian dish. Toasted bread crumbs, not cheese, are the appropriate topping.*

2 medium fennel bulbs, trimmed and sliced

1 cup chopped fresh dill

½ teaspoon saffron threads

½ cup plus 1 tablespoon olive oil

¼ cup plain dry bread crumbs

1 pound fresh sardines, cleaned and filleted (see Note)

Salt and freshly ground black pepper

1 large onion, chopped

6 anchovy fillets

½ cup dried currants

½ cup pine nuts

1 pound perciatelli or bucatini

**1.** Bring at least 4 quarts of water to a boil in a large pot. Add the fennel and dill and cook until tender when pierced with a fork, about 10 minutes. Scoop out the fennel and dill with a slotted spoon, reserving the cooking water. Let the fennel and dill cool, then finely chop them. In a small bowl, soak the saffron threads in 2 tablespoons of the fennel water.

**2.** In a small skillet, heat 1 tablespoon of the oil over medium heat and cook the bread crumbs, stirring constantly, until toasted, about 5 minutes.

**3.** In a large skillet, heat $^1/_4$ cup of the oil. Fry the sardines cut-side down first in the oil until cooked through, about 1 minute on each side. Sprinkle with salt and pepper. Transfer the sardines to a plate.

**4.** Wipe out the skillet. Pour the remaining $^1/_4$ cup of the oil into the skillet. Add the onion and cook over medium heat until golden, about 10 minutes. Add the anchovies, currants, pine nuts, saffron, and salt and pepper to taste. Cook, stirring often, 10 minutes.

**5.** Add the fennel and dill to the onion with one cup of the cooking water. Cook, stirring, 10 minutes.

**6.** Add more water to the pot to equal 4 quarts of water for cooking the pasta. Bring the water to a boil. Add 2 tablespoons of salt, then the pasta. Stir well, gently pushing the pasta down until it is completely covered with water. Cook over high heat, stirring frequently, until the pasta is al dente, tender yet still firm to the bite. Drain the pasta.

**7.** Transfer the pasta to the skillet with the fennel mixture and toss well. Spoon half the pasta into a warm serving bowl. Layer with half of the sardines. Add the remaining pasta. Sprinkle with the bread crumbs and top with the sardines. Serve immediately.

# *Penne with Zucchini, Swordfish, and Herbs*

## *Penne con Zucchine e Pesce Spada*

**Makes 4 to 6 servings**

*This pasta is inspired by one I saw in a favorite Italian cooking magazine, A Tavola ("at the table"), in a story about cooking at a beach house. The zest and herbs make the dish light and fresh. It is perfect on a summer day—even if you're not at the beach—followed by a tomato salad.*

1/4 cup olive oil

12 ounces swordfish, trimmed and cut into 1/2-inch cubes

Salt and freshly ground black pepper

4 to 6 small zucchini, about 1 pound, cut into 1/2-inch pieces

4 green onions, chopped

2 tablespoons chopped fresh rosemary

2 tablespoons chopped fresh chives

1 tablespoon chopped fresh mint

½ teaspoon dried oregano, crumbled

½ teaspoon grated lemon zest

1 pound penne

**1.** In a large skillet, heat 1 tablespoon oil over medium heat. Add the swordfish and cook until the fish loses its pink color, about 5 minutes. Remove the swordfish and transfer to a plate. Sprinkle with salt and pepper.

**2.** Add the remaining 3 tablespoons oil to the pan and heat over medium heat. Add the zucchini, green onions, and salt to taste. Cook, stirring often, until the zucchini are just tender, about 10 minutes.

**3.** Return the swordfish to the pan. Stir in the herbs and lemon zest and remove from the heat.

**4.** Bring at least 4 quarts of water to a boil in a large pot. Add 2 tablespoons of salt, then the pasta. Stir well. Cook over high heat, stirring frequently, until the pasta is al dente, tender yet still firm to the bite. Drain the pasta, reserving some of the cooking water.

**5.** Add the pasta to the skillet and toss over high heat 1 minute to combine. Add some of the reserved pasta water, if needed. Serve immediately.

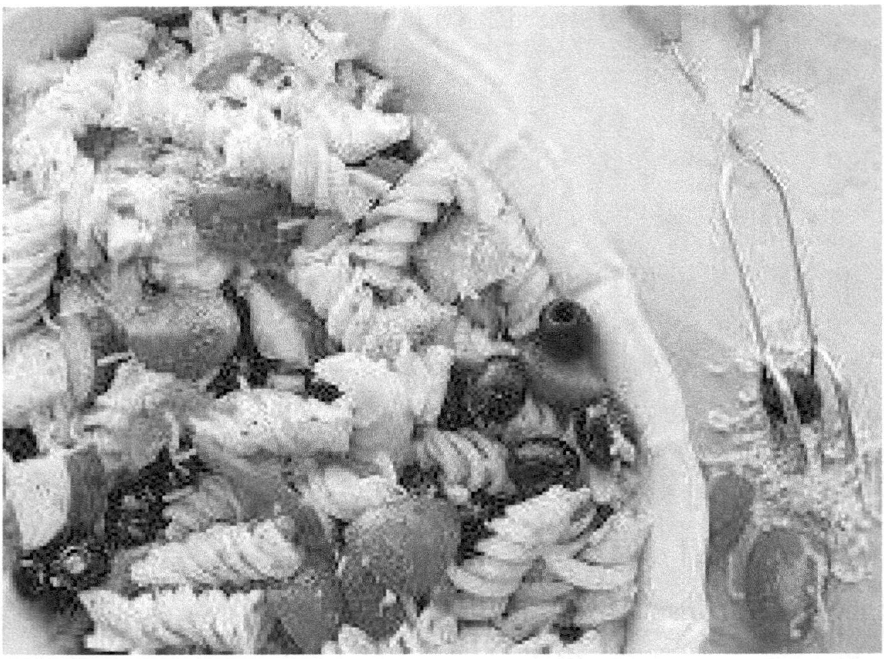

## *Christmas Eve Spaghetti with Baccala*

### *Spaghetti con la Baccala*

**Makes 6 servings**

*Baccala is an important part of the all-fish menu served in most southern Italian homes on Christmas Eve. This recipe was given to me by my aunt, Millie Castagliola, whose family came from Sicily. Aunt Millie makes this same sauce as a filling for a double-crust pizza.*

1 pound stockfish or baccala,

Salt

¼ cup olive oil

2 medium onions, thinly sliced

2 celery ribs, thinly sliced

2 garlic cloves, finely chopped

2 cups chopped canned imported Italian tomatoes with their juice

Pinch of crushed red pepper

½ cup sliced green olives

2 tablespoons capers, rinsed and drained

1 pound spaghetti or linguine

Extra-virgin olive oil

**1.** Bring about 1 quart of water to a boil in a wide saucepan. Add the fish and salt to taste. Reduce the heat to low. Simmer the fish until very tender, about 10 minutes. Remove the fish with a slotted spoon. Let cool slightly. With your fingers, remove any skin and bones. Cut the fish into bite-size pieces.

**2.** Pour the oil into a large saucepan. Add the onions and celery and cook over medium heat until the vegetables are golden, about 15 minutes. Stir in the garlic and cook 2 minutes more.

**3.** Add the tomatoes and red pepper. Cook, stirring occasionally, until the sauce is thick, 20 to 30 minutes.

**4.** Add the fish, olives, and capers and cook 10 minutes. Taste for salt.

**5.** Bring at least 4 quarts of water to a boil in a large pot. Add 2 tablespoons of salt, then the pasta. Stir well, gently pushing the pasta down until it is completely covered with water. Cook, stirring frequently, until the pasta is al dente, tender yet still firm to the bite. Drain the pasta, reserving a little of the cooking water.

**6.** Add the pasta to the pan with the sauce. Toss well over medium heat, adding a little of the cooking water if needed. Drizzle with a little extra– virgin olive oil and serve immediately.

## *Linguine with Tuna Pesto*

## *Linguine al Tonno*

**Makes 4 to 6 servings**

*The uncooked sauce for this Sicilian pasta is similar to pesto, but flavored with anchovies. Just before serving, the sauce and pasta are tossed with canned tuna.*

1 cup tightly packed fresh basil leaves

¾ cup tightly packed fresh parsley leaves

⅓ cup pine nuts

2 medium garlic cloves

1 (2-ounce) can anchovy fillets, drained

⅓ cup extra-virgin olive oil

2 tablespoons fresh lemon juice

1 (7-ounce) can tuna in oil (preferably imported Italian or Spanish tuna in olive oil)

Salt

1 pound linguine

**1.** In a food processor fitted with the steel blade, chop the basil, parsley, pine nuts, and garlic until fine. Add the anchovy fillets, oil, and lemon juice and process until smooth.

**2.** Bring at least 4 quarts of water to a boil in a large pot. Meanwhile, in a large serving bowl, mash the tuna with a fork. Stir in the sauce.

**3.** Add 2 tablespoons of salt, then the pasta, to the boiling water. Stir well, gently pushing the pasta down until it is completely covered with water. Cook the pasta, stirring frequently, until al dente, tender yet still firm to the bite. Drain the pasta, reserving some of the cooking water.

**4.** Transfer the pasta to the bowl with the sauce. Add some of the cooking water and toss well. Serve immediately.

# *Cold Pasta with Vegetable Confetti and Seafood*

## *Pasta Fredda con Verdure e Crostacei*

**Makes 6 to 8 servings**

*On one trip to Italy, the main reason I visited Argenta, a small town in Emilia-Romagna, was to dine at a fine restaurant called Il Trigabolo. The restaurant is closed now, but I still remember my delight when they served me this refreshing cold pasta, crunchy with bits of chopped vegetables and seafood. Most of the vegetables are blanched—that is, they are dropped into the boiling water, then immediately placed under cold water to stop the cooking and cool them. The cool water sets their bright color, and the vegetables keep some of their crunchy texture.*

*Pasta should be rinsed in cool water only in a preparation like this—when you want to stop the cooking and serve the pasta cold.*

1 large firm ripe tomato, cored and diced

1/2 pound cooked small shrimp, cut into 1/4-inch pieces

1 cup chopped cooked lobster or 1/4 pound cooked crabmeat, picked over

1/4 cup snipped fresh chives

¼ cup chopped fresh basil

¼ cup extra-virgin olive oil, plus more for drizzling

Coarse salt and freshly ground black pepper

1 pound thin spaghetti

¾ cup very finely chopped red bell pepper

¾ cup very finely chopped yellow bell pepper

¾ cup very finely chopped zucchini

2 small carrots, cut into matchstick strips

**1.** In a large serving bowl, combine the tomato with the shrimp, lobster, herbs, and olive oil. Season with salt and pepper.

**2.** Bring at least 4 quarts of water to a boil in a large pot. Add 2 tablespoons of salt, then the spaghetti. Stir well, gently pushing the pasta down until it is completely covered with water. Cook over high heat, stirring frequently. About 30 seconds before the pasta is ready, add the peppers, zucchini, and carrots. Stir well. As soon as the pasta is al dente, tender yet still firm to the bite, drain it and the vegetables into a large colander placed in the sink. The vegetables will be just slightly wilted.

**3.** Rinse the pasta and vegetables under cool running water. Drain well.

**4.** Add the pasta to the tomato and seafood mixture. Toss well. Drizzle with additional oil and toss again. Serve immediately.

## *Fresh Egg Pasta*

### *Pasta al Uovo*

**Makes about 1 pound**

*Here is a basic all-purpose pasta dough that I use for fettuccine, lasagne, and ravioli. The dough can be assembled by hand, in a food processor, or in a heavy-duty mixer, and it can be rolled out on a board with a rolling pin or in a pasta rolling machine. If you have never made pasta before, read the recipe through before beginning. The most important thing is to get the balance of flour and eggs right so that the dough is neither sticky nor dry. Because the freshness and size of the eggs and the type and humidity level of the flour vary slightly, it is not possible to give exact proportions.*

*Making fresh pasta is as easy as making any other dough, but it does take some patience. Make it ahead of time, if you like. It keeps well at cool room temperature up to a week, or it can be refrigerated or frozen. A small amount of olive oil helps to keep the dough moist as you work.*

About 2½ cups unbleached all-purpose flour

4 large eggs, beaten

1 teaspoon olive oil (optional, but a good idea, especially for stuffed pastas)

## Preparing the Dough by Hand

**1.** Pour the flour into a mound on a countertop or large pasta board. A rough surface such as wood or plastic is better than a smooth one such as marble or granite. With a fork, make a wide hole in the center of the mound. Pour the eggs and olive oil into the hole and begin stirring with one hand, gradually incorporating some of the flour from the inside of the hole. Use your other hand to support the wall of flour surrounding the eggs, so they don't spill out.

**2.** When the dough forms a ball and becomes too firm to stir, in about 1 minute, sweep the remaining flour to one side. Lightly flour your hands and begin kneading. Push the dough away with the heels of your hands and pull it back toward you with your fingertips. Turn the dough as you are doing this for even kneading. Continue kneading, gradually incorporating some of the remaining flour until the ball becomes somewhat smooth, feels moist, and is only slightly sticky, about 3 minutes. Add only enough flour to create a firm ball of dough, or it may become too dry.

**3.** Put the dough aside for a moment and cover it with an inverted bowl. Wash and dry your hands to remove hardened scraps of dough. Scrape the kneading surface clean with a plastic or metal dough scraper or spatula to remove any hardened pieces of dough and excess flour that might later cause lumps. Throw out the scraps.

**4.** Lightly dust your hands with flour. Resume kneading the dough until it is smooth and elastic, moist yet not sticky, about 8 to 10 minutes. Add more flour if necessary. There should be no streaks of flour on the dough, and the color should be evenly yellow. The more the dough is kneaded, the lighter and more resilient the pasta will be, so do not skimp on kneading. Work quickly so that the dough does not dry out.

**Making the Dough with a Food Processor or Heavy-Duty Mixer**

**1.** Pour the eggs and olive oil into a food processor fitted with the steel blade, or into the bowl of a heavy-duty electric mixer fitted with the flat beater. With the machine running, begin adding the flour a tablespoon at a time. Mix until the dough forms a ball and cleans the inside of the bowl, about 1 minute. Pinch the dough. It should feel moist but not sticky and should be fairly smooth. If not, add more flour as needed.

**2.** Place the dough on a lightly floured surface and knead it for 1 minute, adding more flour if necessary, until it is firm, smooth without streaks of flour, and moist but not sticky.

**Spinach Pasta:** Pasta made with fresh spinach has not only a bright green color but also a good flavor. To make fresh spinach pasta, use 3 cups flour, 3 large eggs, and 1 pound of fresh spinach, cooked, squeezed dry, and very finely chopped (about $^3/_4$ cup cooked spinach). Combine the ingredients as for Fresh Egg Pasta at left. Makes about $1^1/_4$ pounds of pasta.

## Letting the Dough Rest

Whether you have made it by hand or machine, cover the dough with an inverted bowl and let it rest for 30 minutes or up to 2 hours at room temperature.

## Rolling Out the Dough By Hand

**1.** Lightly dust a countertop or large board with flour. Be sure that the surface is perfectly flat and not warped.

**2.** Cut the dough into 2 pieces. It may feel moister after it rests because the eggs have absorbed the flour. While you work with one piece, keep the remainder covered. With your hands, shape one piece of dough into a disk. Choose a wooden rolling pin at least 24 inches long and $1^1/_2$ to 2 inches wide and dust it lightly with flour. Place the pin in the center and push it away from you toward the edge of the dough. Rotate the dough a quarter turn, center the pin on it and push it toward the edge once more. Repeat, rotating the dough and rolling it out from the center, keeping the shape round and the thickness even, until the dough reaches the desired thinness. Flip the dough over from time to time to be sure it is not sticking. If necessary, dust lightly with flour.

**3.** Work quickly so that the dough does not dry out. If it should tear, pinch it together or patch it with a small piece of dough from the edge. The dough is ready when it is very thin and you can easily see your hand through it when it is held up to the light. Roll out the remaining dough in the same way. Be sure to make all of the dough pieces of equal thickness. Turn the pieces often so that they do not stick. If the dough will be used to make stuffed pasta such as ravioli, it should be kept covered so that it remains pliable. Use it as soon as possible.

**4.** Cut the dough into the desired size and shape while it is still soft and pliable. See the various pasta recipes in sections Fresh Pasta, Lasagne, and Stuffed Fresh Pasta for instructions on cutting and shaping the dough.

**Rolling Out the Dough with a Pasta Machine**

1. Following the manufacturer's instructions, clamp the pasta machine to one end of a large countertop or sturdy table. Set the rollers at the widest opening and dust them lightly with flour.

2. Cut the dough into 4 to 6 pieces. It may feel moister after it rests because the eggs have absorbed the flour. While you work with one piece, keep the remainder covered. Flatten one piece of dough into an oval disk. Turn the handle of the pasta machine with one hand while the other guides the piece of dough through the rollers. If the dough sticks or tears, dust it lightly with flour.

3. Remove the dough from the machine and fold it lengthwise into thirds. Pass the dough through the machine again, flouring it if necessary.

4. Close the rollers slightly by moving the dial to the next notch. Pass the dough through the rollers. As the dough emerges, lift it straight out so that it stays flat without wrinkling. Do not fold it.

5. Continue to pass the dough through the machine, moving the dial up one notch each time until the desired thinness is reached. This will vary according to the machine, but I usually stop at the second-to-last setting for fettuccine and flat pasta and the last notch for stuffed pasta. The pasta should be thin enough that you can see your hand through it without tearing. Don't be

tempted to re-roll scraps of dough. Hardened edges can stick in the machine and tear the pasta.

**6.** Lay the strip of dough on a lightly floured kitchen towel. Roll out the remaining dough in the same way. Be sure to make all of the strips of equal thickness. Turn the pieces often so that they do not stick. If the dough will be used to make stuffed pasta such as ravioli, it should be kept covered so that it remains pliable. Use it as soon as possible.

**7.** Cut the dough into the desired size and shape while it is still soft and pliable. See the various pasta recipes in sections Fresh Pasta, Lasagne, and Stuffed Fresh Pasta for instructions on cutting and shaping the dough.

## Making Pasta Noodles

Lasagne, papardelle, fettuccine, tagliatelle, and tagliarini are all flat ribbons of pasta. Their use depends on the type of sauce you are making and regional preferences. Generally, the lighter the sauce, the narrower the pasta.

**1.** Make the pasta as described for Fresh Egg Pasta.

**2.** Let the dough dry until it is slightly leathery but still pliable, about 20 minutes.

**3.** If using your pasta machine's cutting attachment, follow the manufacturer's instructions. Turn the crank with one hand, passing the sheet of dough through the cutters. As the dough emerges, lift it straight out with your other hand so that the strands do not collect on the countertop and become wrinkled.

**4.** If working by hand, first cut the dough into 5-inch lengths for pappardelle and 10-inch lengths for the other pastas. Loosely roll up a strip of dough. With a large heavy chef's knife, cut the rolled up pasta crosswise into strips 3 inches wide for lasagne, 3/4 inches wide for papardelle, 1/3 inch wide for fettuccine, 1/4 inch for tagliatelle, and 1/8 inch for tagliarini. Separate the strips and place them flat on a floured surface to dry about 1 hour at room temperature.

**Storing Fresh Egg Pasta**

Fresh pasta may be used immediately, frozen, or allowed to dry completely. To freeze the pasta, place the strips on baking sheets lightly dusted with flour so that they do not touch. Place the baking sheets in the freezer. When the pasta is firm, gently gather it into a bundle and wrap it well in layers of plastic wrap or foil. Store in the freezer up to one month.

To dry, place the pasta strips, not touching, on baking sheets. Cover each sheet with lightweight cloth kitchen towels. Do not cover them with plastic or foil or they will turn moldy. Leave the strips at room temperature for several days until the pieces are completely dry and snap when broken. Store in plastic bags in the pantry until ready to use.

# *Fettuccine with Butter and Parmigiano*

## *Fettuccine al Burro*

**Makes 4 to 6 servings**

*Even the pickiest children love fresh egg pasta tossed with butter and cheese. Keep in mind that fresh pasta cooks quickly; it will get mushy fast if you walk away.*

6 tablespoons unsalted butter

1 pound fresh fettuccine

Salt

1 cup freshly grated Parmigiano-Reggiano

Freshly ground black pepper

**1.** Melt the butter in a small saucepan and keep warm.

**2.** Bring at least 4 quarts of water to a boil. Add the pasta and salt to taste. Stir well. Cook over high heat, stirring frequently, until the pasta is al dente, tender yet firm to the bite. Drain the pasta, reserving some of the cooking water.

**3.** Pour the pasta into a warm serving bowl. Add half the cheese and toss well. Add the butter and a little of the cooking water if the pasta seems dry. Sprinkle with the remaining cheese and toss again. Sprinkle with freshly ground pepper if desired.

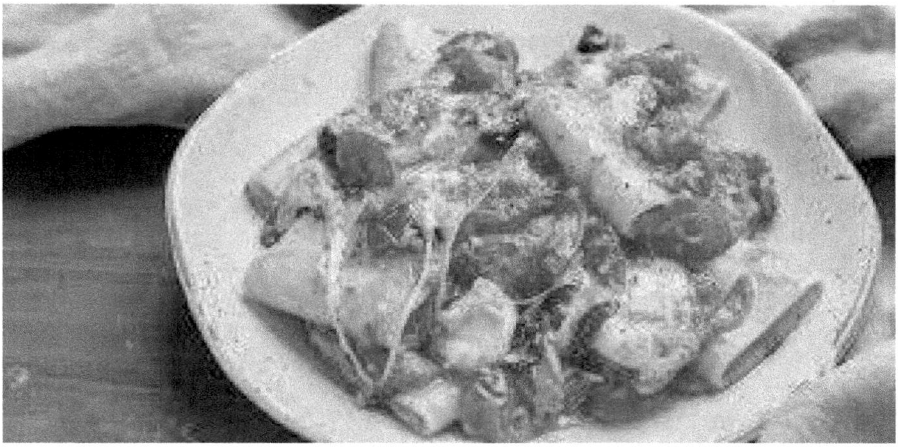

# *Fettuccine with Butter and Cheese*

## *Fettuccine all'Alfredo*

**Makes 6 to 8 servings**

*In the early 1910s Alfredo Di Lelio, whose family owned a trattoria in Rome, created this rich pasta dish of fresh fettuccine, butter, and Parmigiano. The dish became so popular that Alfredo was soon running a bigger, fancier restaurant under his own name, where he would prepare the pasta at tableside, serving it up to diners with great fanfare and a gold fork and spoon. Silent movie stars Douglas Fairbanks, Sr., and his wife, Mary Pickford, were said to have been among the restaurant's many famous patrons.*

*This recipe was given to me by Russell Bellanca, owner of the Alfredo The Original of Rome Restaurants in New York City and Epcot Center, Florida. According to Russell, this is the recipe as developed by Alfredo Di Lelio. His son, Alfredo II, gave it to Russell's dad, who was a business partner many years ago. At Alfredo The Original, the pasta is handmade from a mix of three different flours and organic egg yolks, though I use my own homemade pasta.*

*Serve the pasta in small portions. It is very rich.*

1½ sticks (¾ cup) unsalted butter, at room temperature for at least 30 minutes

1 cup freshly grated Parmigiano-Reggiano, plus more for serving (optional)

1 pound fresh fettuccine

Salt

**1.** In a large bowl with an electric mixer, beat the butter with the cheese until it forms a smooth cream, about 2 minutes.

**2.** Bring at least 4 quarts of water to a boil. Add the pasta and salt to taste. Stir well. Cook over high heat, stirring frequently, until the pasta is al dente, tender yet still firm to the bite. Drain the pasta, reserving a little of the cooking water. Toss the pasta with the butter and cheese and a few tablespoons of the cooking water.

**3.** Serve immediately with additional cheese, if desired.

# *Fettuccine with Spring Vegetables*

## *Fettuccine Primavera*

**Makes 4 to 6 servings**

*This recipe was reportedly invented at Le Cirque Restaurant in New York. Though it has never been on the menu there, regular patrons know that they can request it at any time. Other vegetables can be used, such as peppers, green beans, or zucchini, so feel free to improvise according to what you have on hand.*

4 tablespoons unsalted butter

¼ cup chopped shallots

1 cup chopped carrots

1 cup broccoli florets, cut into bite-size pieces

4 asparagus, trimmed and cut into bite-size pieces

½ cup fresh or frozen peas

1 cup heavy or whipping cream

Salt and freshly ground black pepper

1 pound fresh fettuccine

¾ cup freshly grated Parmigiano-Reggiano

10 basil leaves, stacked and cut into thin ribbons

**1.** In a skillet large enough to hold the fettuccine, melt the butter over medium heat. Add the shallots and carrots and cook, stirring occasionally, five minutes or until softened.

**2.** Bring at least 4 quarts of water to a boil in a large pot. Add salt to taste. Add the broccoli and asparagus and cook for 1 minute. With a slotted spoon, scoop out the vegetables and drain them well, leaving the water boiling in the pot.

**3.** Put the broccoli and asparagus in the skillet along with the peas and cream. Bring to a simmer. Season to taste with salt and pepper. Remove from the heat.

**4.** Put the fettuccine into the boiling water and cook, stirring frequently, until the pasta is al dente, tender yet still firm to the bite. Drain the fettuccine and add it to the skillet. Add the cheese and toss well. Sprinkle with basil and serve immediately.

# *Fettuccine with Gorgonzola Cream*

## *Fettuccine con Crema di Gorgonzola*

**Makes 4 to 6 servings**

*Of all the blue cheeses produced around the world, gorgonzola is my favorite. To make it, cow's milk is innoculated with penicillin spores, which gives the cheese its color and distinct flavor. It is not too sharp and melts beautifully, so it is ideal for sauces. Use a mild type of gorgonzola for this recipe.*

2 tablespoons unsalted butter

8 ounces gorgonzola dolce, rind removed

1 cup heavy or whipping cream

Salt

1 pound fresh fettuccine

Freshly ground black pepper

½ cup freshly grated Parmigiano-Reggiano

**1.** In a medium saucepan, melt the butter and add the gorgonzola. Stir over low heat until the cheese is melted. Stir in the cream.

Bring the sauce to a simmer and cook 5 minutes or until the sauce is slightly thickened.

2. Bring at least 4 quarts of water to a boil. Add the pasta and salt to taste. Stir well. Cook over high heat, stirring frequently, until the pasta is al dente, tender yet still firm to the bite. Drain the pasta, reserving some of the cooking water.

3. In a large warm serving bowl, toss the pasta with the sauce. Add the Parmigiano and toss again. Add a little of the cooking water, if needed, to thin the pasta. Serve immediately.

# *Tagliarini with Pesto, Genoa Style*

## *Tagliarini al Pesto*

**Makes 4 to 6 servings**

*In Liguria in the springtime, thin strands of fresh pasta are served with pesto tossed with slender green beans and sliced new potatoes. The vegetables carry the flavor of the pesto, cut some of the richness, and add texture.*

*The word* pesto *means pounded, and there are several other types of pesto sauces, though this is the best known.*

1 cup packed fresh basil leaves

½ cup packed fresh flat-leaf parsley

¼ cup pine nuts

1 garlic clove

Salt and freshly ground black pepper to taste

⅓ cup extra-virgin olive oil

1 cup freshly grated Parmigiano-Reggiano or Pecorino Romano

4 medium waxy potatoes, peeled and thinly sliced

8 ounces thin green beans, cut into 1-inch lengths

1 pound fresh tagliarini or fettuccine

2 tablespoons unsalted butter, at room temperature

**1.** In a food processor or blender, combine the basil, parsley, pine nuts, garlic, and a pinch of salt. Chop fine. With the machine running, add the oil in a steady stream and process until smooth. Stir in the cheese.

**2.** Bring at least 4 quarts of water to a boil. Add the potatoes and green beans. Cook just until tender, about 8 minutes. Scoop out the vegetables with a slotted spoon. Place them in a warmed serving bowl. Cover and keep warm.

**3.** Add the pasta to the boiling water and stir well. Cook over high heat, stirring frequently, until the pasta is al dente, tender yet still firm to the bite. Drain the pasta, reserving some of the cooking water.

**4.** Add the pasta, pesto, and butter to the serving bowl with the vegetables. Toss very well, adding a little of the cooking water if the pasta seems dry. Serve immediately.

## *Fettuccine with Artichokes*

### *Fettuccine con Carciofi*

**Makes 4 to 6 servings**

*Carts loaded with artichokes appear at the outdoor markets all over Rome in springtime. Their long stems and leaves are still attached, which helps to keep them from drying out. Roman cooks know that the stems are as tasty as the artichoke hearts. They only need peeling and can be cooked right alongside the artichokes or chopped for a stuffing.*

3 medium artichokes

¼ cup olive oil

1 small onion, finely chopped

¼ cup chopped fresh flat-leaf parsley

1 garlic clove, finely chopped

Salt and freshly ground black pepper to taste

½ cup dry white wine

1 pound fresh fettuccine

Extra-virgin olive oil

**1.** Cut off the top $^1/_2$ to $^3/_4$ inch of the artichokes with a large, sharp knife. Rinse artichokes under cold water, spreading the leaves open. Avoid the little thorns on the remaining tips of the leaves. Bend back and snap off all of the dark green leaves until you reach the pale yellowish cone of tender leaves at the center of the artichoke. Peel the tough outer skin around the base and stems. Leave stems attached to the base; trim the ends of stems. Cut artichokes in half lengthwise and scoop out the fuzzy chokes with a spoon. Cut artichokes into thin lengthwise slices.

**2.** Pour oil into a saucepan large enough to hold the cooked pasta. Add onion, parsley, and garlic and cook over medium heat until the onion is golden, about 15 minutes.

**3.** Add artichoke slices, wine, and salt and pepper to taste. Cover and cook until artichokes are tender when pierced with a fork, about 10 minutes.

**4.** Bring at least 4 quarts of water to a boil. Add 2 tablespoons of salt, then the pasta. Stir well. Cook over high heat, stirring frequently, until the pasta is al dente, tender yet still firm to the bite. Drain the pasta, reserving some of the cooking water. Add the pasta to the pan with the artichokes.

**5.** Add a drizzle of extra-virgin olive oil and a little of the reserved cooking water if the pasta seems dry. Toss well. Serve immediately.

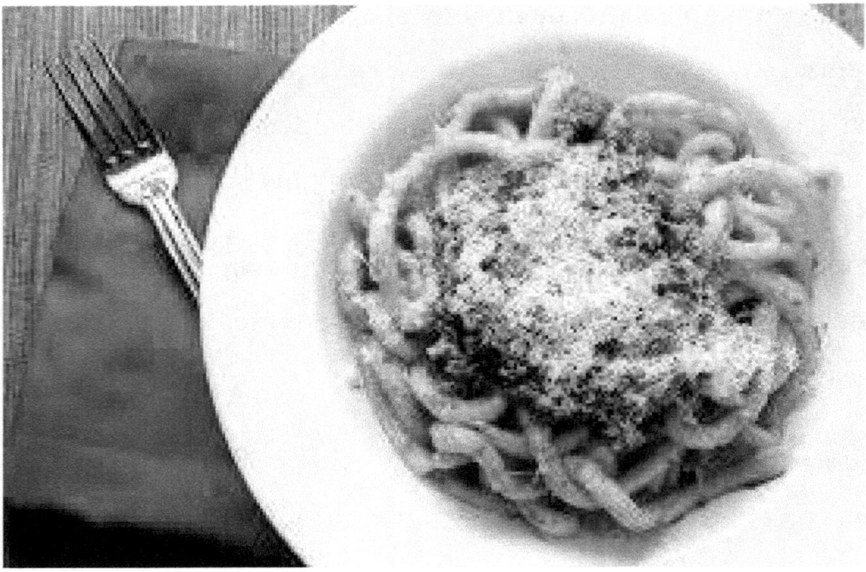

# *Fettuccine with Tomato Fillets*

## *Fettuccine al Filetto di Pomodoro*

**Makes 4 to 6 servings**

*Strips of ripe peeled tomatoes cooked until barely tender are wonderful with fresh fettuccine. The tomatoes retain all of their sweet fresh flavor in this mild sauce.*

4 tablespoons unsalted butter

¼ cup finely chopped onion

1 pound plum tomatoes, peeled and seeded and cut into ½-inch strips

6 fresh basil leaves

Salt to taste

1 pound fresh fettuccine

Freshly grated Parmigiano-Reggiano

**1.** In a large skillet, heat 3 tablespoons of the butter over medium-low heat until melted. Add the onion and cook until golden, about 10 minutes.

**2.** Stir in the tomato fillets, basil leaves, and a couple of pinches of salt. Cook until the tomatoes are tender, about 5 to 10 minutes.

**3.** Bring at least 4 quarts of water to a boil. Add 2 tablespoons of salt, then the pasta. Stir well. Cook over high heat, stirring frequently, until the pasta is al dente, tender yet still firm to the bite. Drain the pasta, reserving some of the cooking water.

**4.** Add the fettuccine to the skillet along with the remaining 1 tablespoon of butter. Toss well. Add a little of the cooking water if the pasta seems dry. Serve immediately with the cheese.

# *Fettuccine with a Thousand Herbs*

## *Fettuccine alle Mille Erbe*

**Makes 4 to 6 servings**

*This is one of my favorite summer pastas, one that I love to make when the herbs in my garden are in full bloom and the tomatoes are perfectly ripe. The recipe comes from the Locanda dell'Amorosa, a restaurant and inn located in Sinalunga in Tuscany. There they used* stracci, *meaning "raggedy," a shape of pasta similar to pappardelle cut with a fluted pastry wheel so that the edges are jagged. Fettuccine are a good substitute.*

*There is a lot of chopping involved in making this sauce, but it can be done well in advance of serving. Do not substitute dried herbs for the fresh. Their flavor would be too aggressive in this pasta. The more varieties of herbs that you use, the more complex the flavor will be, but even if you don't use all of the varieties listed, it will still be delicious.*

¼ cup chopped Italian parsley

¼ cup chopped fresh basil

¼ cup chopped fresh tarragon

2 tablespoons chopped fresh mint

2 tablespoons chopped fresh marjoram

2 tablespoons chopped fresh thyme

8 fresh sage leaves, finely chopped

1 sprig fresh rosemary, finely chopped

⅓ cup extra-virgin olive oil

Salt and freshly ground black pepper

1 pound fresh fettuccine

½ cup freshly grated Pecorino Romano

2 medium ripe tomatoes, peeled, seeded, and chopped

**1.** In a bowl large enough to contain all of the ingredients, combine the herbs, olive oil, and salt and pepper to taste. Set aside.

**2.** Bring at least 4 quarts of water to a boil. Add 2 tablespoons of salt, then the pasta Stir well. Cook over high heat, stirring frequently, until the pasta is al dente, tender yet still firm to the bite. Drain the pasta, reserving some of the cooking water.

3. Add the pasta to the bowl with the herb mixture and toss well. Add the cheese and toss again. Scatter the tomatoes over the pasta and serve immediately.

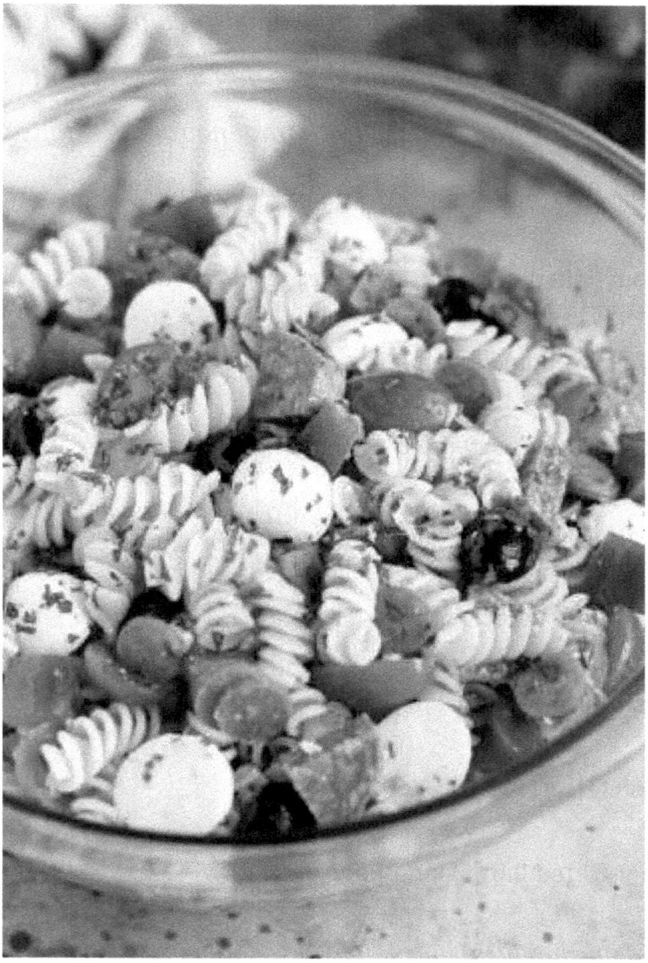

# *Fettuccine with Sausage and Cream*

## *Fettuccine con Salsiccia*

**Makes 4 to 6 servings**

*Roasted red peppers, bits of sausage, and green peas get tangled among the creamy fettuccine for great flavor in every bite in this recipe from Emilia-Romagna. Try to find meaty pork sausages without a lot of spices for this recipe.*

8 ounces plain Italian pork sausages, casings removed

1 cup heavy or whipping cream

½ cup diced drained roasted red peppers

½ cup fresh or frozen tiny peas

1 tablespoon chopped fresh flat-leaf parsley

Salt and freshly ground black pepper

1 pound fresh fettuccine

½ cup freshly grated Parmigiano-Reggiano

**1.** Heat a large skillet over medium heat. Add the sausage and cook, stirring often to break up any lumps, until no longer pink, about 5 minutes. Remove the meat to a cutting board, let cool a little, then chop finely.

**2.** Wipe out the skillet. Pour the cream and the chopped sausage into the pan and bring it to a simmer. Stir in the roasted peppers, peas, parsley, and salt and pepper to taste. Cook 3 minutes or until the peas are tender. Turn off the heat.

**3.** Bring at least 4 quarts of water to a boil. Add 2 tablespoons of salt, then the pasta. Stir well. Cook over high heat, stirring frequently, until the pasta is al dente, tender yet still firm to the bite. Drain the pasta, reserving some of the cooking water.

**4.** Toss the pasta in the pan with the sauce. Add the cheese and toss again. Stir in a little of the cooking water, if necessary. Serve immediately.

# *Green and White Pasta with Sausage and Cream*

## *Paglia e Fieno*

**Makes 4 to 6 servings**

*Paglia e Fieno literally translates as "straw and hay," the whimsical name in Emilia-Romagna for this dish of thin green and white noodles cooked together. They are typically dressed with a creamy sausage sauce.*

2 tablespoons unsalted butter

8 ounces plain Italian pork sausage, casings removed and chopped fine

1 cup heavy cream

½ cup fresh or frozen tiny peas

Salt

½ pound fresh egg tagliarini

½ pound fresh spinach tagliarini

Freshly ground black pepper

½ cup freshly grated Parmigiano-Reggiano

1. In a skillet large enough to hold the cooked pasta, melt the butter over medium heat. Add the sausage meat and cook, stirring frequently, just until the meat is no longer pink, about 5 minutes. Do not brown.

2. Stir in the cream and peas and bring to a simmer. Cook 5 minutes or until the cream is slightly thickened. Remove from the heat.

3. Bring at least 4 quarts of water to a boil. Add 2 tablespoons of salt, then the pasta. Stir well. Cook over high heat, stirring frequently, until the pasta is al dente, tender yet still firm to the bite. Drain the pasta, reserving some of the cooking water.

4. Stir the pasta into the sausage mixture. Add a generous grind of black pepper and the cheese and toss thoroughly. Serve immediately.

## *Fettuccine with Leeks and Fontina*

### *Fettuccine con Porri e Fontina*

**Makes 4 to 6 servings**

*The finest fontina cheese comes from the Valle d'Aosta in northwestern Italy. It has a creamy texture and an earthy flavor reminiscent of truffles. It is a perfect eating cheese, and it melts well.*

4 medium leeks

½ cup water

2 tablespoons unsalted butter

Salt

¾ cup heavy cream

4 ounces sliced imported Italian prosciutto, cut crosswise into thin strips

Freshly ground black pepper

1 pound fresh fettuccine

1 cup grated Fontina Valle d'Aosta or Asiago

**1.** Trim away the green tops and root ends of the leeks. Cut them in half lengthwise and rinse well under cold running water, getting any grit out from between the layers. Drain the leeks and cut them into thin crosswise slices. There should be about $3^1/_2$ cups of sliced leeks.

**2.** In a skillet large enough to hold the pasta, combine the leeks, water, butter, and salt to taste. Bring the water to a simmer and cook over low heat until the leeks are tender and slightly translucent and most of the liquid has evaporated, about 30 minutes.

**3.** Add the cream and simmer 2 minutes more or until slightly thickened. Stir in the prosciutto and some pepper. Remove the sauce from the heat.

**4.** Bring at least 4 quarts of water to a boil. Add 2 tablespoons of salt, then the pasta. Stir well. Cook over high heat, stirring frequently, until the pasta is al dente, tender yet still firm to the bite. Drain the pasta, reserving some of the cooking water.

**5.** Add the pasta to the skillet with the sauce and toss well. Add a little cooking water if the pasta seems dry. Add the fontina, toss again, and serve.

## *Fettuccine with Mushrooms and Prosciutto*

### *Fettuccine con Funghi e Prosciutto*

**Makes 4 to 6 servings**

*Prosciutto is normally sliced paper-thin, but when adding it to a cooked dish, I often prefer to have the meat cut into a single thick slice, which I then cut into narrow strips. It holds its shape better and doesn't overcook when exposed to heat.*

4 tablespoons unsalted butter

1 package (10 ounces) mushrooms, thinly sliced

1 cup frozen peas, partly thawed

Salt and freshly ground black pepper

4 ounces imported Italian prosciutto, in one slice about ¼ inch thick, cut crosswise into thin strips

1 pound fresh fettuccine

½ cup heavy cream

½ cup freshly grated Parmigiano-Reggiano

**1.** In a skillet large enough to hold all of the ingredients, melt the butter over medium heat. Add the mushrooms and cook, stirring occasionally, until the mushroom juices evaporate and the mushrooms begin to brown, about 10 minutes.

**2.** Stir in the peas. Sprinkle with salt and pepper and cook 2 minutes. Stir in the prosciutto and turn off the heat. Cover to keep warm.

**3.** Bring at least 4 quarts of water to a boil. Add 2 tablespoons of salt, then the pasta. Stir well. Cook over high heat, stirring frequently, until the pasta is al dente, tender yet still firm to the bite. Drain the pasta, reserving some of the cooking water.

**4.** Transfer the pasta to the skillet with the vegetables and prosciutto. Turn the heat to high. Add the cream and cheese and toss again. Add some of the cooking water if the pasta seems dry. Serve immediately.

## *Summer Tagliatelle*

### *Tagliatelle Estiva*

**Makes 4 to 6 servings**

*Everything about this pasta is sweet and fresh, from the disks of small, fresh zucchini, to the sunny ripe flavor of the tomatoes, to the creamy mild flavor of the ricotta salata cheese. This pressed, firm, dry form of ricotta is used both as a table cheese and for grating. Substitute a mild pecorino or Parmigiano-Reggiano if you cannot find this kind of ricotta.*

1 small onion, chopped

¼ cup olive oil

3 very small zucchini, cut into ¼-inch disks

Salt

2 cups grape tomatoes, halved lengthwise

1 cup torn basil leaves

1 pound fresh spinach fettuccine

½ cup grated ricotta salata

**1.** In a large skillet, cook the onion in the oil over medium heat 5 minutes. Add the zucchini and salt to taste. Cook 5 minutes or until softened. Stir in the tomatoes and cook 5 minutes more or until the zucchini are tender. Stir in half of the basil and turn off the heat.

**2.** Meanwhile, bring at least 4 quarts of water to a boil. Add 2 tablespoons of salt, then the pasta. Stir well. Cook, stirring often, until the pasta is al dente, tender yet still firm to the bite.

**3.** Drain the pasta and toss it with the sauce. Add the cheese and remaining 1/2 cup of the basil and toss again. Serve immediately.

# *Fettuccine with Mushroom and Anchovy Sauce*

## *Fettuccine al Funghi*

**Makes 4 to 6 servings**

*Even those who don't ordinarily enjoy anchovies will appreciate the flavor boost they give to this sauce. Their presence isn't obvious; the anchovies melt into the sauce.*

2 large garlic cloves, finely chopped

⅓ cup olive oil

12 ounces white or brown-white mushrooms, very thinly sliced

Salt and freshly ground black pepper

½ cup dry white wine

6 anchovy fillets, chopped

2 large fresh tomatoes, peeled, seeded, and chopped, or 1½ cups chopped canned imported Italian tomatoes, with their juice

1 pound fresh fettuccine

¼ cup chopped fresh flat-leaf parsley

2 tablespoons unsalted butter

**1.** In a skillet large enough to hold all of the pasta, cook the garlic in the oil over medium heat for 1 minute.

**2.** Add the mushrooms and cook, stirring often, until the liquid evaporates and the mushrooms begin to brown, about 10 minutes. Stir in the wine and bring to a simmer.

**3.** Add the anchovies and tomatoes. Reduce the heat to low and cook 10 minutes.

**4.** Bring at least 4 quarts of water to a boil. Add 2 tablespoons of salt, then the pasta. Stir well. Cook over high heat, stirring frequently, until the pasta is al dente, tender yet still firm to the bite. Drain the pasta, reserving some of the cooking water.

**5.** Transfer the pasta to the skillet with the sauce and toss well with the parsley. Add the butter and toss again, adding a little of the cooking water if needed. Serve immediately.

## *Fettuccine with Scallops*

### *Fettuccine con Canestrelli*

**Makes 4 to 6 servings**

*I usually make this pasta with large sea scallops. They are plump and sweet and available all year round. Smaller bay scallops, available primarily in the northeast in the summer time, are excellent too. Do not confuse them with the tasteless calico scallops that come from warm waters. They are sometimes passed off as bay scallops, though they are generally much smaller and lacking in flavor. Bay scallops are about a half-inch in diameter, with a creamy white color, while the calicos are about a quarter of an inch in size and very white.*

4 large garlic cloves, finely chopped

¼ cup olive oil

1 pound sea scallops, cut into ½-inch pieces, or bay scallops, left whole

Pinch of crushed red pepper

Salt

1 large ripe tomato, seeded and diced

2 cups fresh basil leaves, torn into 2 or 3 pieces

1 pound fresh fettuccine

**1.** In a skillet large enough to hold all the pasta, cook the garlic in the oil over medium heat until the garlic is lightly golden, about 2 minutes. Stir in the scallops, pepper, and salt to taste. Cook just until the scallops are opaque, about 1 minute.

**2.** Stir in the tomato and basil. Cook 1 minute until the basil is slightly wilted. Remove the skillet from the heat.

**3.** Bring at least 4 quarts of water to a boil. Add 2 tablespoons of salt, then the pasta. Stir well. Cook over high heat, stirring frequently, until the pasta is al dente, tender yet still firm to the bite. Drain the pasta, reserving some of the cooking water.

**4.** Add the pasta to the skillet. Toss well, adding some of the cooking water if needed. Serve immediately.

## *Tagliarini with Shrimp and Caviar*

### *Tagliarini al Gamberi e Caviale*

**Makes 4 to 6 servings**

*Coral-colored salmon caviar is a delicious counterpoint to the sweetness of the shrimp and creamy sauce on this pasta. I came up with this recipe several years ago for an Italian New Year's Eve feast for the Washington Post.*

12 ounces medium shrimp, peeled and deveined, cut into ½-inch pieces

1 tablespoon unsalted butter

2 tablespoons vodka or gin

1 cup heavy cream

Salt and freshly ground white pepper

2 tablespoons very finely chopped green onion

½ teaspoon fresh lemon zest

1 pound fresh tagliarini

3 ounces salmon caviar

1. In a skillet large enough to hold all of the pasta, melt the butter over medium heat. Add the shrimp and cook, stirring, until pink and almost cooked through, about 2 minutes. With a slotted spoon, remove the shrimp to a plate.

2. Add the vodka to the skillet. Cook, stirring, until the liquid evaporates, about 1 minute. Add the cream and bring to a simmer. Cook until the cream thickens slightly, about one minute more. Stir in the shrimp and a pinch of salt and pepper. Add the green onion and lemon zest. Remove from the heat.

3. Bring at least 4 quarts of water to a boil. Add 2 tablespoons of salt, then the pasta. Cook, stirring frequently, until the pasta is al dente, tender yet still firm to the bite. Drain the pasta, reserving a little of the cooking water.

4. Pour the pasta into the skillet with the sauce and toss well over medium heat. Add a little of the cooking water if the pasta seems dry. Divide the pasta among the plates. Top each portion with a spoonful of caviar and serve immediately.

## *Crisp Pasta with Chickpeas, Puglia Style*

### *Ceci e Tria*

**Makes 4 servings**

*Short strips of fresh pasta are sometimes called* tria *in Puglia and elsewhere in southern Italy. In the tenth century, the Norman ruler of Sicily, Roger II, had an Arabic geographer prepare a survey of his kingdom. The geographer, al-Idrisi, wrote that he saw people making food from flour in the form of threads that they called by the Arabic word for string,* itriyah. *The shortened form,* tria, *is still used.*

*Tria are about as wide as fettuccine, but they are cut into 3-inch lengths. The pasta in this recipe is given an unusual treatment: Half is boiled in the normal way, but the other half is fried until it becomes crisp, like the noodles you find in Chinese restaurants. The two are combined in a tasty chickpea sauce. This is a traditional recipe from the southern part of Puglia, near Lecce. It is unlike any other pasta recipe I have tried in Italy.*

3 tablespoons plus ½ cup olive oil

1 small onion, chopped

1 celery rib, chopped

1 garlic clove, finely chopped

$1\frac{1}{2}$ cups cooked or canned chickpeas, drained

1 cup peeled, seeded, and chopped tomato

2 tablespoons finely chopped fresh flat-leaf parsley

2 cups water

Salt and freshly ground black pepper

12 ounces fresh fettuccine, cut into 3-inch lengths

**1.** In a large saucepan combine the 3 tablespoons olive oil and the onion, celery, and garlic. Cook over medium heat until softened, about 5 minutes. Add the chickpeas, tomato, parsley, and water. Season to taste with salt and pepper. Bring to a simmer and cook 30 minutes.

**2.** Set out a tray covered with paper towels. In a large skillet, heat the remaining $^{1}/_{2}$ cup oil over medium heat. Add one fourth of the pasta and cook, stirring, until it blisters and begins to brown lightly, about 4 minutes. Remove the pasta with a slotted spoon and drain it on the tray. Repeat with another quarter of the pasta.

**3.** Bring at least 4 quarts of water to a boil. Add 2 tablespoons of salt, then the rest of the pasta. Stir well. Cook over high heat, stirring frequently, until the pasta is al dente, tender yet still firm to the bite. Drain the pasta, reserving some of the cooking water.

**4.** Stir the boiled pasta into the simmering sauce. Stir in some of the cooking water if the pasta seems dry. It should resemble a thick soup.

**5.** Add the fried pasta to the pan and stir. Serve immediately.

# *Tagliarini with Abruzzese Chocolate Ragù*

## *Pasta Abruzzese al Cioccolato Amaro*

**Makes 4 to 6 servings**

*I adapted this recipe from one that my friend Al Bassano told me he had gotten from an Italian language website. I was intrigued because I had never seen or tasted anything like it before. I couldn't wait to try it, and I was not disappointed. A small amount of chocolate and cinnamon adds a subtle richness to the sauce.*

*The original recipe called for serving the ragù with* chitarrina, *a typically Abruzzese-style egg pasta made on a device known as a* chitarra, *or "guitar." The guitar in this case is a simple wooden frame strung with a row of guitar strings. A sheet of fresh pasta dough is laid across the strings and a rolling pin is rolled over the dough. The taut strings cut the dough into square spaghetti-like strands. Tagliarini are a good substitute for the chitarrina.*

1 medium onion, finely chopped

¼ cup olive oil

8 ounces ground pork

Salt and freshly ground black pepper

½ cup dry red wine

1 cup tomato puree

¼ cup tomato paste

1 cup water

1 tablespoon chopped bittersweet chocolate

½ teaspoon sugar

Pinch of ground cinnamon

1 pound fresh tagliarini

1. In a medium saucepan, cook the onion in the oil over medium heat until the onion is tender and golden, about 10 minutes. Add the pork and cook, crumbling the meat with the back of a spoon, until lightly browned. Season with salt and pepper to taste.

2. Add the wine and bring to a simmer. Cook until most of the wine has evaporated.

3. Stir in the tomato puree, tomato paste, and water. Turn the heat to low and cook 1 hour, stirring occasionally, until the sauce is thick.

**4.** Stir in the chocolate, sugar, and cinnamon until the chocolate is melted. Taste for seasoning.

**5.** Bring at least 4 quarts of water to a boil. Add 2 tablespoons of salt, then the pasta. Stir well. Cook over high heat, stirring frequently, until the pasta is al dente, tender yet still firm to the bite. Drain the pasta, reserving some of the cooking water.

**6.** In a large warm serving bowl, toss the pasta with the sauce. Add a little of the reserved cooking water if needed. Serve immediately.

# *Bologna-Style Lasagne*

## *Lasagne Bolognese*

**Makes 8 to 10 servings**

*This lasagne from Bologna in northern Italy is altogether different from the southern Italian version that follows this recipe, though both are classics. The Bolognese verison is made with green-tinted spinach lasagne rather than egg lasagne, and the only cheese used is Parmigiano-Reggiano, while the southern version has mozzarella, ricotta, and Pecorino Romano. Creamy white béchamel sauce is a standard ingredient in the northern variety, while the southern version contains much more meat. Try them both—they're equally delicious.*

3 to 4 cups Bologna-Style Ragù

3 cups Béchamel Sauce

1 pound fresh spinach lasagne

Salt

1½ cups freshly grated Parmigiano-Reggiano

2 tablespoons unsalted butter

**1.** Prepare the two sauces. Bring at least 4 quarts of water to a boil. Have ready a large bowl of cold water. Add to the boiling water half the lasagne and 2 tablespoons of salt. Cook until the pasta is tender but slightly underdone. Remove the pasta with a slotted spoon and place it in the cold water. Cook the remaining lasagne strips the same way. Lay the cooled lasagne sheets out flat on lint free towels.

**2.** Butter a 13 × 10 × 2–inch pan. Set aside the 2 best-looking pasta strips for the top layer. Set aside 1/2 cup of the béchamel and 1/4 cup of the cheese. Make a layer of pasta, overlapping the pieces. Spread with thin layers of the béchamel, then the ragu, then the cheese. Repeat the layering, ending with the pasta. Spread the top layer with the reserved 1/2 cup of béchamel. Sprinkle with the reserved 1/4 cup cheese. Dot with the butter. (If you are making the lasagne ahead of time, cover tightly with plastic wrap and refrigerate overnight.)

**3.** Place a rack in the center of the oven. Preheat the oven to 375°F. Bake the lasagne 45 minutes. If the lasagne is browning too much, cover it loosely with foil. Bake 15 minutes more or until the sauce is bubbling and a knife inserted in the center comes out warm. Let stand 15 minutes before serving.

# *Neapolitan Lasagne*

## *Lasagne Napolitana*

**Makes 8 to 10 servings**

*Whenever I make lasagne, I can't help but think of my favorite Italian children's fable,* Pentolin delle Lasagne, *written by A. Rubino and published in the children's section of the newspaper* Corriere della Sera *in 1932. It is the story of a man who always wore on his head a* pentolino di terracotta, *a clay pot for cooking lasagne. He felt that it protected him from the elements, and he was always ready to make lasagne on a moment's notice. Not surprisingly, he was the best lasagne maker in his country of Pastacotta ("cooked pasta"), though people laughed at him because of his silly headgear. Thanks to his lasagne pot and a bit of magic, he saved the citizens of Pastacotta from a famine, became king, and lived happily ever after, making lasagne every Sunday for everyone in his kingdom.*

*This is lasagne the way my mother made it, and my grandmother before her. It is incredibly rich, but absolutely irresistible.*

About 8 cups Neapolitan Ragù, made with tiny meatballs

Salt

1 pound fresh lasagne

2 pounds whole or part-skim ricotta

1¼ cups freshly grated Pecorino-Romano

1 pound fresh mozzarella, thinly sliced

**1.** Prepare the ragù. Remove the meat pieces, meatballs, and sausages from the sauce. Set aside the pork and veal for another meal. Cut the sausages into thin slices and set them aside with the meatballs for the lasagne.

**2.** Lay out some lint-free kitchen towels on a flat surface. Have ready a large bowl of cold water.

**3.** Bring about 4 quarts of water to a boil. Add 2 tablespoons of salt. Add the lasagne a few pieces at a time. Cook the lasagne until tender but slightly underdone. Scoop the pasta out of the water. Place the cooked pasta in the cold water. When cool enough to handle, lay the pasta sheets out flat on the towels. The towels can be stacked one on top of the other. Continue cooking and cooling the remaining lasagne in the same way.

**4.** In a 13 × 9 × 2–inch pan, spread a thin layer of the sauce. Make a layer of pasta, overlapping the pieces slightly. Spread with 2 cups of the ricotta, then the tiny meatballs and sliced sausages, then the mozzarella. Spoon on about 1 cup more of the sauce and sprinkle with $^1/_4$ cup of the grated cheese.

**5.** Repeat the layers, ending with pasta, sauce, and grated cheese. (If you are making the lasagne ahead of time, cover tightly with plastic wrap and refrigerate overnight.)

**6.** Place a rack in the center of the oven. Preheat the oven to 375°F. Bake the lasagne 45 minutes. If the lasagne is browning too much, cover it loosely with foil. Bake 15 minutes more or until the top is browned and the sauce is bubbling around the edges.

**7.** Remove the lasagne from the oven and let set 15 minutes. Cut the lasagne into squares and serve.

# *Spinach and Mushroom Lasagne*

## *Lasagne di Funghi e Spinaci*

**Makes 8 to 10 servings**

*Parma is heaven for pasta lovers. Wrapped around tasty fillings, tossed with sauces, or layered with different ingredients, the pasta there seems light as air and always delicious. This dish is based on my recollection of a heavenly creamy lasagne I ate in Parma many years ago.*

3 cups Béchamel Sauce

1 pound fresh spinach, trimmed

Salt

5 tablespoons unsalted butter

1 small onion, finely chopped

1½ pounds button mushrooms, chopped

1 pound fresh lasagne

1½ cups freshly grated Parmigiano-Reggiano

1. Prepare the béchamel sauce. Then, place the spinach in a large pot with 1/2 cup of water. Add a pinch of salt. Cover and cook over medium heat until the spinach is tender, about 5 minutes. Drain the spinach well. Let cool. Wrap the spinach in a towel and squeeze it to extract as much of the juice as possible. Chop the spinach and set it aside.

2. In a large skillet, melt four tablespoons of the butter over medium heat. Add the onion and cook, stirring occasionally, until softened, about 5 minutes.

3. Stir in the mushrooms and salt and pepper to taste. Cook, stirring frequently, until all of the liquid evaporates and the mushrooms are tender. Stir in the chopped cooked spinach.

4. Set aside 1/2 cup of the béchamel sauce. Stir the remainder into the vegetable mixture.

5. Have ready a large bowl of cold water. Lay out some lint-free kitchen towels on a work surface.

6. Bring a large pot of water to a boil. Add 2 tablespoons of salt. Add the lasagne a few pieces at a time. Cook the lasagne until tender but slightly underdone. Scoop the pasta out of the water. Place the cooked pasta in the cold water. When cool enough to handle, lay the pasta sheets out flat on the towels, which can be

stacked one on top of the other. Continue cooking and cooling the remaining lasagne in the same way.

**7.** Butter a 13 × 9 × 2–inch pan. Set aside the 2 best-looking pasta strips for the top layer. Make a layer of pasta in the prepared pan, overlapping the pieces. Spread with a thin layer of the vegetables and a sprinkle of cheese. Repeat the layering, ending with the pasta. Spread with reserved béchamel. Sprinkle with the remaining cheese. Dot with the remaining butter.

**8.** Preheat the oven to 375°F. Bake 45 minutes. If the lasagne is browning too much, cover it loosely with foil. Bake 15 minutes more or until the top is browned and the sauce is bubbling around the edge. Remove from the oven and let stand 15 minutes before serving. Cut into squares to serve.

# *Green Lasagne*

## *Lasagne Verde*

**Makes 8 to 10 servings**

*Green lasagne noodles are layered with ham, mushrooms, tomatoes, and béchamel sauce. To make this meatless, just eliminate the ham.*

3 cups Béchamel Sauce

1 ounce dried porcini mushrooms

2 cups hot water

4 tablespoons unsalted butter

1 tablespoon olive oil

1 garlic clove, finely chopped

12 ounces white mushrooms, chopped

½ teaspoon dried marjoram or thyme

Salt and freshly ground black pepper

1 cup peeled, seeded, and chopped fresh tomatoes or canned imported Italian tomatoes, drained and chopped

8 ounces sliced boiled ham, chopped

1¼ cups freshly grated Parmigiano-Reggiano

1¼ pounds green lasagne

**1.** Prepare the béchamel sauce. Put the dried mushrooms in the water and let soak 30 minutes. Remove the mushrooms from the bowl and reserve the liquid. Rinse the mushrooms under cold running water to remove any grit, paying special attention to the ends of the stems where soil collects. Chop the mushrooms coarsely. Strain the mushroom liquid through a paper coffee filter into a bowl.

**2.** In a large skillet, melt two tablespoons of the butter with the oil over medium heat. Add the garlic and cook one minute. Add the fresh and dried mushrooms, marjoram, and salt and pepper to taste. Cook, stirring occasionally, for 5 minutes. Add the tomatoes and reserved mushroom liquid and cook until thickened, about 10 minutes more.

**3.** Have ready a large bowl of cold water. Lay out some lint-free kitchen towels on a work surface.

**4.** Bring at least 4 quarts of water to a boil. Add 2 tablespoons of salt. Add the lasagne a few pieces at a time. Cook the lasagne until tender but slightly underdone. Scoop the pasta out of the water. Place the cooked pasta in the cold water. When cool enough to handle, lay the pasta sheets out flat on the towels, which can be stacked one on top of the other. Continue cooking and cooling the remaining lasagne in the same way.

5. Butter a 13 × 9 × 2–inch pan. Set aside the 2 best-looking pasta strips for the top layer. Set aside 1/2 cup of the béchamel and 1/4 cup of the cheese. Make a layer of pasta, overlapping the pieces. Spread with a thin layer of the béchamel, mushroom sauce, ham, and cheese. Repeat the layering, ending with the pasta. Spread with reserved béchamel. Sprinkle with the remaining cheese. Dot with the remaining butter.

6. Place a rack in the center of the oven. Preheat the oven to 375°F. Bake the lasagne 45 minutes. If the lasagne is browning too much, cover it loosely with foil. Uncover and bake 15 minutes more or until the top is browned and the sauce is bubbling around the edges. Let stand 15 minutes before serving. Cut into squares to serve.

# *Green Lasagne with Ricotta, Basil, and Tomato Sauce*

## *Lasagne Verde con Ricotta, Basilico, e Marinara*

**Makes 8 to 10 servings**

*My grandmother always made the Neapolitan-style lasagne, but once in a while she would surprise us with this meatless version, especially in the summer when a typical meat ragù seemed too heavy.*

*Just thinking about this lasagne makes me hungry. The fragrance of the basil, the richness of the cheese, and the sweetness of the tomato sauce is a combination that I find tantalizing. It is a beautiful dish, too, with its layers of red, green, and white.*

5 to 6 cups Marinara Sauce or Fresh Tomato Sauce

Salt and freshly ground black pepper

1¼ pounds fresh green lasagne

2 pounds fresh part-skim ricotta

1 egg, slightly beaten

1 cup freshly grated Parmigiano-Reggiano or Pecorino Romano

8 ounces fresh mozzarella cheese, thinly sliced

1 large bunch basil, stacked and cut into narrow ribbons

**1.** Prepare the sauce, if necessary. Then, have ready a large bowl of cold water. Lay out some lint-free kitchen towels on a work surface.

**2.** Bring at least 4 quarts of water to a boil. Add 2 tablespoons of salt. Add the lasagne a few pieces at a time. Cook the lasagne until tender but slightly underdone. Scoop the pasta out of the water. Place the cooked pasta in the cold water. When cool enough to handle, lay the pasta sheets out flat on the towels, which can be stacked one on top of the other. Continue cooking and cooling the remaining lasagne in the same way.

**3.** In a bowl, beat the ricotta, egg, and salt and pepper to taste.

**4.** In a 13 × 9 × 2–inch pan, spread a thin layer of the sauce. Place two of the lasagne in the pan in a single layer, overlapping slightly. Spread evenly with half of the ricotta mixture, and sprinkle with 2 tablespoons of the grated cheese. Arrange one third of the mozzarella slices on top.

**5.** Make a second layer of lasagne and spread it with sauce. Scatter the basil on top. Layer with the cheeses as described above. Repeat for a third layer. Make a final layer of lasagne, sauce, mozzarella, and grated cheese. (Can be made ahead to this point. Cover with plastic wrap and refrigerate several hours or overnight.)

**6.** Place a rack in the center of the oven. Preheat the oven to 375°F. Bake the lasagne for 45 minutes. If the lasagne is browning too much, cover it loosely with foil. Bake 15 minutes more or until the top is browned and the sauce is bubbling around the edges. Let stand 15 minutes. Cut into squares and serve.

# *Eggplant Lasagne*

## *Lasagne con la Parmigiana*

**Makes 8 to 10 servings**

*My friend Donatella Arpaia, who spent childhood summers with her family in Italy, remembers a favorite aunt who would make lasagne with fresh vegetables early in the morning to bring to the beach for lunch later in the day. The pan was carefully wrapped in towels, and the contents would still be warm when they sat down to eat.*

*This version resembles eggplant Parmesan, with the addition of fresh lasagne noodles. It is perfect for a summer buffet or to serve vegetarians.*

2 medium eggplants (about 1 pound each)

Salt

Olive oil

1 medium onion, finely chopped

5 pounds fresh plum tomatoes, peeled, seeded, and chopped, or 2 (28-ounce) cans imported Italian peeled tomatoes, drained and chopped

Freshly ground black pepper

2 tablespoons chopped fresh flat-leaf parsley

2 tablespoons chopped fresh basil

1 pound fresh lasagne

1 pound fresh mozzarella, quartered and cut into thin slices

1 cup freshly grated Parmigiano-Reggiano

**1.** Trim the eggplants and cut them into thin slices. Sprinkle the slices with salt and layer them in a colander set over a plate. Let stand at least 30 minutes. Rinse the eggplant in cold water and pat dry.

**2.** Place a rack in the center of the oven. Preheat the oven to 400°F. Generously brush the eggplant slices on both sides with oil. Arrange the slices on large baking sheets. Bake the eggplants 30 minutes, or until tender and lightly browned.

**3.** In a large saucepan, cook the onion in $^1/_3$ cup of olive oil over medium heat, stirring, until tender but not browned, about 10 minutes. Add the tomatoes and salt and pepper to taste. Bring to a simmer and cook until slightly thickened, about 15 to 20 minutes. Stir in the basil and parsley.

**4.** Lay out some lint-free kitchen towels on a work surface. Have ready a large bowl of cold water. Bring at least 4 quarts of water to a boil. Add 2 tablespoons of salt. Cook the lasagne strips a couple of pieces at a time. Remove the strips after one minute, or when they are still firm. Place them in the bowl of water to cool. Then lay them out flat on the towels. Repeat, cooking and cooling the remaining pasta in the same way; the towels can be stacked one on top of the other.

**5.** Lightly oil a 13 × 9 × 2–inch lasagne pan. Spread a thin layer of the sauce in the pan.

**6.** Make a layer of pasta, slightly overlapping the pieces. Spread with a thin layer of sauce, then eggplant slices, mozzarella, and grated cheese. Repeat the layering, ending with pasta, tomato sauce, and grated cheese. (Can be made up to 24 hours in advance. Cover with plastic wrap and refrigerate. Remove from the refrigerator about 1 hour before baking.)

**7.** Preheat the oven to 375°F. Bake 45 minutes. If the lasagne is browning too much, cover it loosely with foil. Bake 15 minutes more or until the top is browned and the sauce is bubbling around the edges. Remove from the oven and let stand 15 minutes before serving. Cut into squares to serve.

# *Ricotta and Ham Cannelloni*

## *Cannelloni al Prosciutto*

**Makes 8 servings**

*Ricotta means "recooked." This fresh cheese is made in Italy from either cow's or sheep's milk whey, the watery liquid left after making a firm cheese, such as pecorino. When the whey is heated, the residual solids coagulate. After draining, the curds are transformed into the soft cheese we know as ricotta. Italians eat it as a breakfast or dessert cheese and in many pasta dishes. This is a southern Italian style cannelloni filled with ricotta and slivers of prosciutto. Any of the tomato sauces can be used with this pasta, but if you prefer a richer dish, you can substitute a meat ragù.*

1 recipe Fresh Egg Pasta, cut into 4-inch squares for cannelloni

1 recipe (about 3 cups) Fresh Tomato Sauce or Tuscan Tomato Sauce

Salt

1 pound fresh mozzarella

1 (16-ounce) container whole or part-skim ricotta

½ cup chopped imported Italian prosciutto (about 2 ounces)

1 large egg, beaten

¾ cup freshly grated Parmigiano-Reggiano

Freshly ground black pepper

**1.** Prepare the pasta and sauce. Lay out some lint-free kitchen towels on a flat surface. Have ready a large bowl of cold water. Bring about 4 quarts of water to a boil. Add salt to taste. Add the pasta squares a few pieces at a time. Cook the pasta until tender but slightly underdone. Scoop the pasta out of the water and place it in the cold water. When cool enough to handle, lay the pasta sheets out flat on the towels, which can be stacked one on top of the other. Continue cooking and cooling the remaining pasta in the same way.

**2.** In a large bowl, combine the mozzarella, ricotta, prosciutto, egg, and 1/2 cup of the Parmigiano. Mix well and add salt and pepper to taste.

**3.** Spoon a thin layer of sauce in the bottom of a large baking dish. Spread about 2 tablespoons of the filling on one end of each pasta square. Roll up the pasta, starting with the filled end, and place the rolls seamside down in the prepared pan.

4. Spoon a thin layer of sauce over the pasta. Sprinkle with the remaining Parmigiano.

5. Place a rack in the center of the oven. Preheat the oven to 375°F. Bake 30 minutes or until the sauce is bubbling and the cheeses are melted. Serve hot.

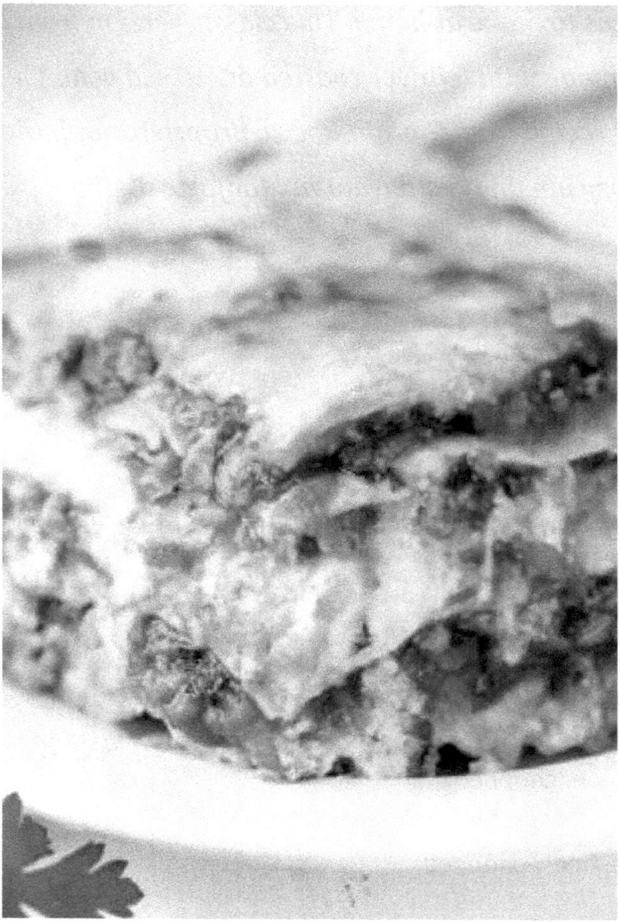

# *Veal and Spinach Cannelloni*

## *Cannelloni di Vitello e Spinaci*

**Makes 8 servings**

*Cannelloni always seem so elegant, yet they are one of the easiest stuffed pastas to make at home. This classic version from Piedmont is typically made with leftover roasted or stewed veal. This is my version of a recipe from Giorgio Rocca, proprietor of Il Giardino da Felicin, a cozy inn and restaurant in Monforte d'Alba.*

3 to 4 cups Béchamel Sauce

1 pound fresh spinach

2 tablespoons unsalted butter

2 pounds boneless veal, cut into 2-inch pieces

2 medium carrots, chopped

1 tender celery rib, chopped

1 medium onion, chopped

1 garlic clove, finely chopped

Salt and freshly ground black pepper

Pinch of freshly ground nutmeg

1½ cups freshly grated Parmigiano-Reggiano

1½ pounds Fresh Egg Pasta, cut into 4-inch squares for cannelloni

**1.** Prepare the béchamel sauce.

**2.** Put the spinach in a large pot over medium heat with ¼ cup of water. Cover and cook 2 to 3 minutes or until wilted and tender. Drain and cool. Wrap the spinach in a lint-free cloth and squeeze out as much water as possible. Finely chop the spinach.

**3.** In a large skillet, melt the butter over medium-low heat. Add the veal, carrots, celery, onion, and garlic. Season to taste with salt and pepper and a pinch of nutmeg. Cover and cook, stirring occasionally, until the meat is very tender, about 1 hour. If the meat becomes dry, add a little water. Let cool. On a cutting board with a large knife, or in a food processor, chop the mixture very fine. Scrape the meat and spinach into a bowl and add 1 cup of the béchamel and 1 cup of the Parmigiano. Mix well and taste for seasoning.

**4.** Meanwhile, prepare the pasta. Lay out some lint-free kitchen towels on a flat surface. Have ready a large bowl of cold water. Bring about 4 quarts of water to a boil. Add 2 tablespoons of salt.

Add the pasta squares a few pieces at a time. Cook the pasta until tender but slightly underdone. Scoop the pasta out of the water and place it in the cold water. When cool enough to handle, lay the pasta sheets out flat on the towels, which can be stacked one on top of the other. Continue cooking and cooling the remaining pasta in the same way.

**5.** Spoon half of the remaining béchamel in a thin layer in a large baking pan. Spread about two tablespoons of the filling on one end of each pasta square and roll up, starting from the filled end. Place the pasta roll seam-side down in the prepared pan. Repeat with the remaining pasta and filling, arranging the rolls close together in the pan. Spoon on the remaining sauce and sprinkle with the remaining 1/2 cup of Parmigiano. (Can be made up to 24 hours in advance. Cover with plastic wrap and refrigerate. Remove from the refrigerator about 1 hour before baking.)

**6.** Place a rack in the center of the oven. Preheat oven to 375°F. Bake 30 minutes or until the cannelloni are heated through and lightly golden. Serve hot.

# *Green and White Cannelloni*

## *Cannelloni alla Parmigiana*

**Makes 8 servings**

*If you visit the Emilia-Romagna region, be sure to stop in Parma. This elegant little city, the birthplace of the great conductor Arturo Toscanini, is renowned for its fine cooking. Many of the city's buildings are painted a sunny yellow color, known as Parma gold. Parma has many fine restaurants where you can taste superb hand-rolled pasta, aged Parmigiano-Reggiano, and the finest balsamic vinegar. I ate these cannelloni at Angiol d'Or, a classic Parma restaurant.*

1 pound Fresh Spinach Pasta, cut into 4-inch squares for cannelloni

2 cups Béchamel Sauce

8 ounces fresh spinach, trimmed

Salt

1 pound whole or part-skim ricotta

2 large eggs, lightly beaten

1½ cups freshly grated Parmigiano-Reggiano

$^1/_4$ teaspoon freshly grated nutmeg

Freshly ground black pepper

4 ounces Fontina Valle d'Aosta, coarsely grated

**1.** Prepare pasta and béchamel sauce. Put the spinach in a large pot over medium heat with $^1/_4$ cup of water. Cover and cook 2 to 3 minutes or until wilted and tender. Drain and cool. Wrap the spinach in a lint-free cloth and squeeze out as much water as possible. Finely chop the spinach.

**2.** Lay out some lint-free kitchen towels on a flat surface. Have ready a large bowl of cold water. Bring about 4 quarts of water to a boil. Add 2 tablespoons salt. Add the pasta squares a few pieces at a time. Cook the pasta until tender but slightly underdone. Scoop the pasta out of the water and place it in the cold water. When cool enough to handle, lay the pasta sheets out flat on the towels, which can be stacked one on top of the other. Continue cooking and cooling the remaining pasta in the same way.

**3.** Stir together the spinach, ricotta, eggs, $^1/_2$ cup of the Parmigiano, the nutmeg, and salt and pepper to taste. Stir in the fontina.

**4.** Place a rack in the center of the oven. Preheat the oven to 375°F. Butter a 13 × 9 × 2–inch baking dish.

**5.** Spread about 1/4 cup of the filling at one end of each pasta square. Roll up the pasta, starting with the filled end. Place the cannelloni seamside down in the pan.

**6.** Spread the sauce over the pasta. Sprinkle with the remaining 1 cup of Parmigiano. Bake 20 minutes or until lightly browned.

# *Cannelloni with Tarragon and Pecorino*

## *Cannelloni di Ricotta al Dragoncello*

**Makes 6 servings**

*Tarragon, with its mild licorice flavor, is not used much in Italy, except occasionally in Umbria and Tuscany. Fresh tarragon is essential for this recipe, since dried tarragon would be too assertive. If you cannot find the fresh tarragon, substitute fresh basil or parsley.*

*These Umbrian-style cannelloni are made with a sheep's milk cheese, such as Pecorino Romano, but Parmigiano-Reggiano can be substituted. Despite the cheese, nuts, and pasta, these cannelloni seem light as air.*

½ recipe (about 8 ounces) Fresh Egg Pasta, cut into 4-inch squares for cannelloni

Salt

1 pound whole or part-skim ricotta

½ cup freshly ground Pecorino Romano, or substitute Parmigiano-Reggiano

1 egg, beaten

1 tablespoon chopped fresh tarragon or basil

¼ teaspoon ground nutmeg

2 tablespoons unsalted butter

¼ cup extra-virgin olive oil

¼ cup pine nuts

1 tablespoon tarragon or basil

Freshly ground black pepper

2 tablespoons freshly grated Pecorino Romano

**1.** Prepare the pasta. Bring at least 4 quarts of water to a boil. Add half the pasta and salt to taste. Stir gently. Cook over high heat, stirring frequently, until the pasta is tender but slightly underdone. Use a slotted spoon to remove the pasta. Transfer the pasta to a bowl of cold water. Cook the remaining pasta in the same way.

**2.** In a large bowl, stir together the cheeses, egg, tarragon, and nutmeg.

**3.** Place a rack in the center of the oven. Preheat the oven to 350° F. Butter a large baking dish.

**4.** Drain a few of the pasta squares on lint-free towels. Spread about 2 tablespoons of the filling in a line at one at one end of each pasta square. Roll up the pasta, starting with the filled end, and place it seam-side down in the pan. Repeat with the remaining pasta and filling.

**5.** In a small saucepan over medium heat, melt the butter with the olive oil. Stir in the pine nuts, tarragon, and pepper. Spoon the sauce over the cannelloni. Sprinkle with the cheese.

**6.** Bake the cannelloni 20 to 25 minutes or until the sauce is bubbling. Let rest 5 minutes before serving.

## *Cheese Ravioli with Fresh Tomato Sauce*

### *Ravioli alla Ricotta*

**Makes 8 servings**

*Cookware stores sell all kinds of ravioli-making equipment. I have a metal traylike contraption that impresses pasta sheets with a series of bellies to hold the filling, then flips over to seal and cut out the perfect ravioli in two sizes. I have handsome brass and wood stamps that I bought in Parma to cut out squares and circles. Then there is the clever wooden rolling pin that cuts out ravioli if you press down on it with the strength of Hercules, and the ravioli cutter that came with my hand-cranked pasta machine. Though I have tried them all, I never use any of them. The simplest way to make ravioli is by hand with minimal equipment. A wavy-edge pastry wheel gives them a pretty border, though you can also cut them with a sharp knife or pizza wheel. They may not be perfect in appearance, but that is part of their homemade charm, and no one has ever complained about their flavor.*

*This is a basic recipe for cheese-filled ravioli the way it is made in many regions of Italy.*

1 pound whole or part-skim ricotta

4 ounces fresh mozzarella, coarsely grated or very finely chopped

1 large egg, beaten

1 cup freshly grated Parmigiano-Reggiano or Pecorino Romano

2 tablespoons chopped fresh parsley

Salt and freshly ground black pepper to taste

4 cups Fresh Tomato Sauce

1 pound Fresh Egg Pasta, rolled out and cut into 4-inch strips

**1.** Mix together the ricotta, mozzarella, egg, $^1/_2$ cup of the Parmigiano, the parsley, and the salt and pepper to taste. Cover and refrigerate.

**2.** Prepare the sauce and pasta. Dust 2 or 3 large baking sheets with flour. Set out a small bowl filled with cool water.

**3.** Lay a strip of the dough on a lightly floured surface. Fold it lengthwise in half to mark the center, then unfold it. Beginning about 1 inch from one of the short ends, place teaspoonfuls of the filling about 1 inch apart in a straight row down one side of the fold. Lightly brush around the filling with the cool water. Fold the dough over the side with filling. Press out any air bubbles and seal the edges. Use a fluted pastry wheel or a sharp knife to cut between the dough-covered mounds of filling. Separate the ravioli and press the edges firmly with the back of a fork to seal. Place the ravioli in a single layer on a baking sheet.

**4.** Repeat with the remaining dough and filling. Cover with a towel and refrigerate until ready to cook, or up to 3 hours, turning the pieces several times so that they do not stick to the pan. (To store them longer, freeze the ravioli on the baking sheets until firm. Place them in a heavy-duty plastic bag and seal tightly. Store in the freezer up to one month. Do not thaw before cooking.)

**5.** Just before serving, bring about 4 quarts of water to a boil in a large pot. Meanwhile, in a medium pot, heat the sauce over low heat. Pour some of the sauce into a heated serving bowl.

**6.** Lower the heat under the pasta pot so that the water boils gently. Add the ravioli and cook until tender, 2 to 5 minutes depending on the thickness of the ravioli and whether or not they were frozen. Scoop the ravioli out of the pot with a slotted spoon. Drain well.

**7.** Place the ravioli in the serving bowl. Pour on the remaining sauce. Sprinkle with the remaining 1/2 cup cheese and serve immediately.

# *Parma-Style Spinach and Cheese Ravioli*

## *Tortelli alla Parmigiana*

**Makes 8 servings**

*While ricotta-filled ravioli are probably the most popular in Italy, a similar version with cooked greens is a favorite also. Spinach or Swiss chard are the most commonly used greens, but escarole, dandelion, beet greens, and borage are also used, depending on the region.*

*In this recipe from Parma, mascarpone is substituted for some of the ricotta, and Swiss chard is the typical green. At one time, it was traditional to serve these for Saint John's Day, June 21st. Note that the Parmigiani call these* tortelli.

1 pound fresh spinach or Swiss chard, stems removed

Salt

1 cup whole or part-skim ricotta

1 cup mascarpone (or an additional cup of ricotta)

1 large egg, beaten

1 cup freshly grated Parmigiano-Reggiano

Pinch of freshly ground nutmeg

Freshly ground black pepper

1 recipe Fresh Egg Pasta, rolled out and cut into 4-inch strips

8 tablespoons (1 stick) unsalted butter

**1.** Place the greens in a large pot with 1/2 cup water and salt to taste. Cover and cook over medium-low heat until the vegetable is wilted and tender, about 5 minutes. Drain and let cool. Wrap the greens in a lint-free kitchen towel or a piece of cheesecloth and squeeze it with your hands to extract all of the juice. Finely chop the greens.

**2.** In a large bowl, stir together the chopped greens, ricotta, mascarpone if using, the egg, 1/2 cup of the grated cheese, nutmeg, and salt and pepper to taste.

**3.** Prepare the pasta. Make and cook the ravioli as described in the recipe for Cheese Ravioli, steps 2 to 6.

**4.** While the ravioli are cooking, melt the butter over medium heat. Pour half of the butter into a serving bowl. Add the ravioli and the remaining melted butter.

**5.** Sprinkle with the remaining $^1/_2$ cup Parmigiano and serve immediately.

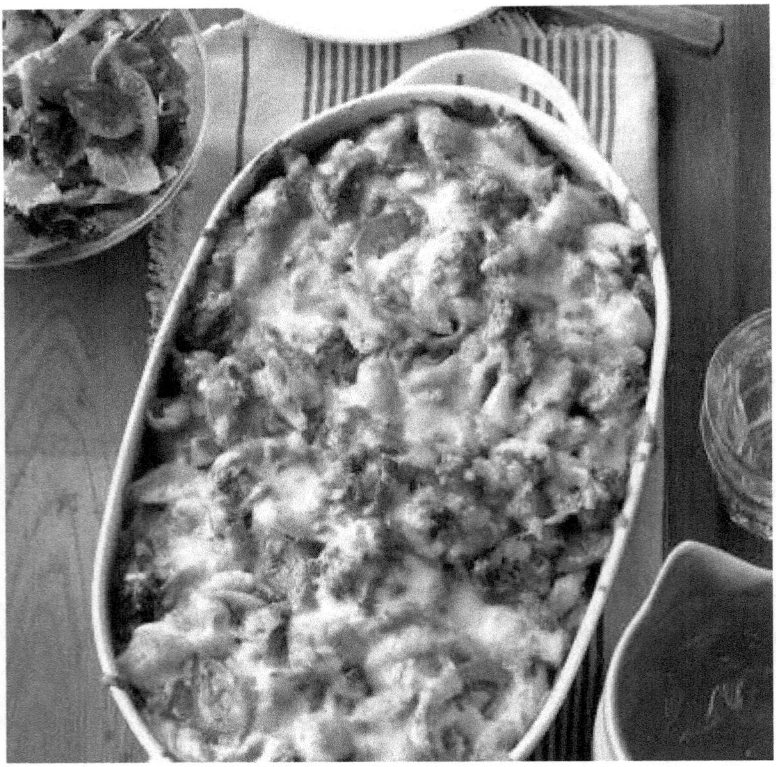

# *Winter Squash Ravioli with Butter and Almonds*

## *Tortelli di Zucca al Burro e Mandorle*

**Makes 8 servings**

*In the fall and winter when winter squashes are plentiful in the market, cooks in Lombardy and Emilia-Romagna make these slightly sweet ravioli accented with the almond flavor of amaretti cookies. The recipe is very old, probably dating back to the Renaissance, when sweet foods often appeared during a meal on aristocratic tables as a sign of wealth.*

*Some recipes call for adding a spoonful of drained, finely chopped* mostarda*—fruits preserved in a tangy mustard syrup—to the squash mixture. Toasted almonds add a nice crunch to the topping.*

About 2 pounds butternut or Hubbard squash

1¼ cup freshly grated Parmigiano-Reggiano

¼ cup finely crushed amaretti cookies

1 large egg

¼ teaspoon ground nutmeg

Salt to taste

1 pound Fresh Egg Pasta, rolled out and cut into 4-inch strips

1 stick (4 ounces) unsalted butter

2 tablespoons chopped toasted almonds

**1.** Place a rack in the center of the oven. Preheat the oven to 400°F. Oil a small baking pan. Cut the squash in half and scoop out the seeds and fibers. Place the halves cut-side down in the pan. Bake 1 hour or until tender when pierced with a knife. Let cool.

**2.** Scrape the flesh away from the skin. Pass the flesh through a food mill fitted with the fine blade or puree it in a food processor or blender. Stir in 3/4 cup of the cheese, the amaretti, egg, nutmeg, and salt. Taste for seasoning.

**3.** Prepare the pasta. Make and cook the ravioli as described in the recipe for Cheese Ravioli, steps 2 to 6.

**4.** While the ravioli are cooking, melt the butter over medium heat. Pour half of the butter into a warm serving bowl. Add the ravioli and the remaining melted butter. Toss them with almonds. Sprinkle with the remaining 1/2 cup cheese. Serve immediately.

# *Meat Ravioli with Tomato Sauce*

## *Agnolotti in Salsa di Pomodoro*

**Makes 8 to 10 servings**

*Italian cooks rarely start from scratch when making a meat filling for fresh pasta. Typically, leftovers from a stew or roast are chopped up and moistened with the meat juices. Cheese, cooked vegetables, or breadcrumbs may be added to extend the filling, and the mixture is bound together with beaten eggs. Because I don't always have leftovers available for ravioli filling, I make this easy stew as a filling for ravioli.*

3 cups Tuscan Tomato Sauce

2 tablespoons unsalted butter

1 pound ground veal or beef

1 boneless skinless chicken breast, cut into 1-inch pieces

1 medium onion, chopped

1 medium carrot, chopped

1 small celery rib, chopped

1 garlic clove, finely chopped

Salt and freshly ground black pepper

½ cup dry white wine

1 cup Parmigiano-Reggiano or Pecorino Romano

2 large egg yolks

1 pound Fresh Egg Pasta, rolled out and cut into 4-inch strips

**1.** Prepare the sauce. Then, melt the butter in a large skillet over medium heat. Add the meat and chicken and cook until the meat loses its pink color, breaking up the lumps of ground meat with a spoon.

**2.** Add the onion, carrot, celery, and garlic. Cook 10 minutes, stirring often, or until the vegetables are softened. Season to taste with salt and pepper.

**3.** Add the wine and simmer 1 minute. Cover the pan and reduce the heat to low. Cook 1½ hours or until the meat is very tender. Add a little water to the pan if the mixture becomes too dry. Remove from the heat and let cool.

**4.** Scrape the meat mixture into a food processor or a food grinder. Chop or grind the meat until it is finely ground, but not pasty. Transfer the meat mixture to a bowl.

**5.** Add 1/2 cup of the grated cheese to the meat mixture and mix well. Taste for seasoning. Stir in the egg yolks.

**6.** Prepare the pasta. Make and cook the ravioli as described in the recipe for <u>Cheese Ravioli</u>, steps 2 to 6. Serve hot with the sauce and sprinkle with remaining 1/2 cup of the cheese.

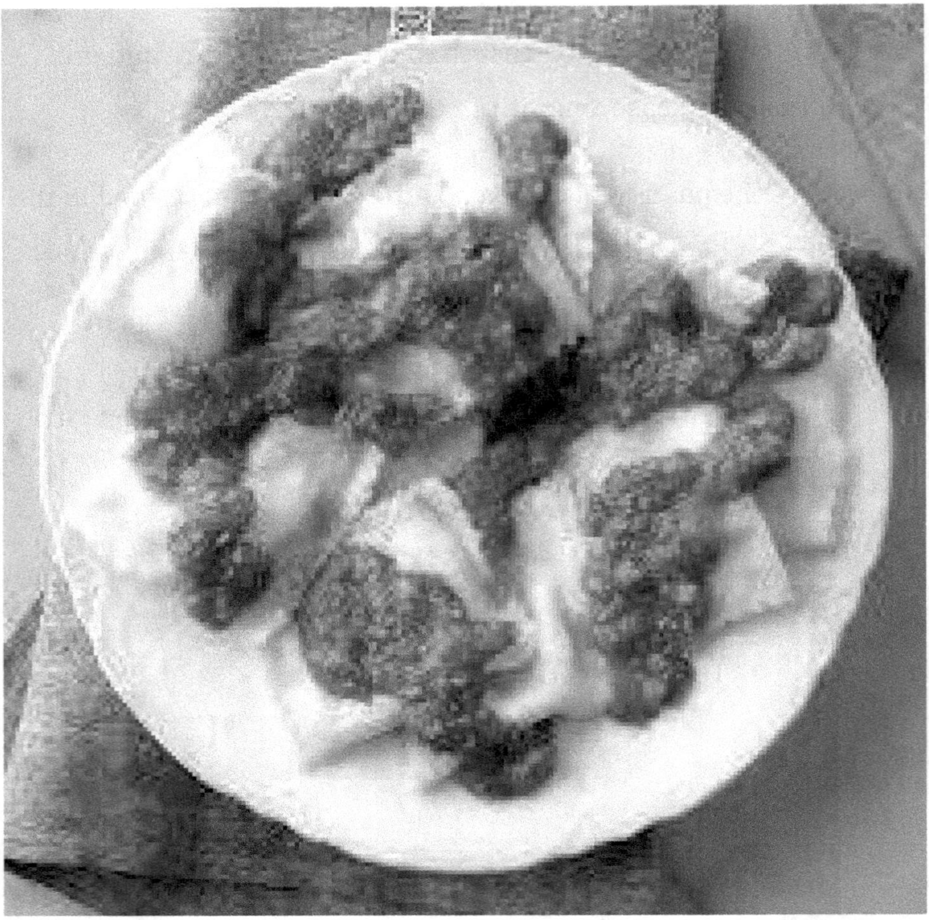

# *Tuscan Sausage Ravioli*

## *Tortelli Casentinese*

**Makes 8 servings**

Tortelli *is another name for ravioli that is used frequently in Tuscany and Emilia-Romagna. These tortelli, stuffed with pork sausage, are made in the style of the Casentino section of Tuscany, a region that is also known for its beautiful wool products.*

3 cups Tuscan Tomato Sauce

1 garlic clove, very finely chopped

2 tablespoons olive oil

1 pound plain Italian pork sausage, skinned

2 large eggs

2 tablespoons tomato paste

1 cup freshly grated Pecorino Romano

¼ cup plain dry bread crumbs

2 tablespoons chopped fresh flat-leaf parsley

Pinch of freshly grated nutmeg

Salt and freshly ground black pepper

1 pound Fresh Egg Pasta, rolled out and cut into 4-inch strips

1. Prepare the sauce. Then, in a large skillet, cook the garlic in the oil over medium heat for 1 minute. Add the sausage meat and cook, stirring frequently, until the meat is just cooked through. Transfer the sausage meat to a cutting board and chop fine.

2. In a large bowl, beat the eggs until blended. Beat in the tomato paste. Stir in the sausage meat, 1/2 cup of the cheese, bread crumbs, nutmeg, and salt and pepper to taste.

3. Prepare the pasta. Make and cook the ravioli as described in the recipe for Cheese Ravioli, steps 2 to 6. Spoon on the sauce and serve immediately with the remaining 1/2 cup grated cheese.

# *Spiced Ravioli, Marches Style*

## *Ravioli Marchegiana*

**Makes 8 servings**

*Cooks in the Marches region on the Adriatic coast, are known for their deft use of spices in savory dishes. These ravioli, for example, made with a variety of vegetables and cheese, are flavored with lemon zest, cinnamon, and nutmeg. Serve them with Marches-Style Ragù or a simple Butter and Sage Sauce.*

About 4 cups Marches-Style Ragù

12 ounces assorted greens such as spinach, Swiss chard, chicory, or dandelion

1 cup whole or part-skim ricotta

1 large egg, beaten

1 cup grated Parmigiano-Reggiano

1 teaspoon grated lemon zest

Pinch of grated nutmeg

Pinch of ground cinnamon

Salt and freshly ground black pepper

1 pound Fresh Egg Pasta, rolled out and cut into 4-inch strips

**1.** Prepare the ragù. Then, put the spinach in a large pot over medium heat with 1/4 cup of water. Cover and cook for 2 to 3 minutes or until wilted and tender. Drain and cool. Wrap the spinach in a lint-free cloth and squeeze out as much water as possible. Finely chop the spinach.

**2.** In a large bowl, mix together the ricotta, egg, 1/2 cup of the cheese, the lemon zest, nutmeg, cinnamon, and salt and pepper to taste.

**3.** Prepare the pasta. Make and cook the ravioli as described in the recipe for Cheese Ravioli, steps 2 to 6. Transfer ravioli to a serving bowl. Spoon on the sauce and serve immediately with the remaining 1/2 cup of cheese.

# *Mushroom Ravioli in Butter and Sage Sauce*

## *Agnolotti ai Funghi*

**Makes 8 servings**

*The combination of mushrooms and marjoram is typical of Liguria, where this recipe originates. White button mushrooms are fine as the stuffing for these ravioli, but for extra-special flavor add some wild mushrooms to the filling.*

3 tablespoons unsalted butter

1 tablespoon olive oil

1 pound fresh mushrooms, sliced thin

1 teaspoon fresh marjoram or thyme or a pinch of dried

Salt and freshly ground black pepper

½ cup whole or part-skim ricotta

1 cup freshly grated Parmigiano-Reggiano

1 egg yolk

1 pound Fresh Egg Pasta, rolled out and cut into 4-inch strips

$^{1}/_{2}$ cup Butter and Sage Sauce

**1.** In a large skillet, melt the butter with the oil over medium heat. Add the mushrooms, marjoram, and salt and pepper to taste. Cook, stirring occasionally, until the mushrooms are tender and the juices have evaporated. Let cool.

**2.** Scrape the mushrooms into a food processor and chop finely. Add the ricotta and $^{1}/_{2}$ cup of the Parmigiano and taste for seasoning. Stir in the egg yolk.

**3.** Prepare the pasta. Make and cook the ravioli as described in the recipe for Cheese Ravioli, steps 2 to 6.

**4.** Meanwhile, make the sauce. Pour half the sauce into a warm serving bowl. Add the cooked ravioli. Spoon on the remaining sauce, and sprinkle with the remaining $^{1}/_{2}$ cup of Parmigiano-Reggiano. Serve immediately.

## *Giant Ravioli with Truffle Butter*

### *Ravioloni al Tuorlo d'Uovo*

**Makes 4 servings**

*One of these extra-large and extra-rich ravioli is sufficient for a first course serving. I first had these years ago at San Domenico Restaurant in Imola, founded by the great chef Nino Bergese, known for his creative approach to classic Italian cooking.*

*This is a most unusual recipe. The fresh egg pasta is filled with a ring of ricotta piped around an egg yolk. When the raviolo is cut, the lightly cooked yolk oozes out and blends with the butter sauce. At San Domenico, the ravioloni were topped with thinly shaved fresh white truffles. The heat of the pasta and sauce brought out their flavor and aroma. The effect was extraordinary, and I will always remember it as one of the most delicious things I have ever eaten.*

*Though they may seem a little tricky, these ravioli really are quite simple to make and very impressive to serve. For best results, assemble the ravioli just before cooking. You can substitute freshly shaved flakes of Parmigiano-Reggiano for the truffle. Most truffle oils have an artificial flavor, so I avoid them.*

1 pound Fresh Egg Pasta, rolled out and cut into four 8 × 4–inch strips

1 cup whole or part-skim ricotta

2 tablespoons freshly grated Parmigiano-Reggiano

Pinch of ground nutmeg

Salt and freshly ground black pepper

4 large eggs

½ cup unsalted butter, melted

Fresh white or black truffle or a large piece of Parmigiano-Reggiano

**1.** Prepare the pasta. Then, mix together the ricotta and grated cheese, nutmeg, and salt and pepper to taste. Scrape the filling into a pastry bag fitted with a ½-inch tip or a heavy-duty plastic bag, cutting off one corner to create a ½-inch opening.

**2.** Keeping the remaining pasta covered, lay out one strip on a countertop. Fold the strip in half crosswise, then unfold to crease the center. Leaving a ½-inch border all around, pipe a circle of the cheese mixture on the pasta to one side of the crease. Separate one egg, setting the white aside for another use. Carefully drop the yolk into the center of the circle. Lightly brush around the cheese with cool water. Fold the other half of the pasta over the filling. With a fork, press the edges of the pasta together to seal. Repeat with the remaining pasta and filling.

**3.** Bring at least 2 quarts of water to a boil. Lower the heat until the water is simmering. Add salt to taste. Carefully place the ravioli in the water and cook just until the pasta is tender, about 3 minutes.

**4.** Spoon a little of the butter into each of 4 warm serving dishes. Remove the ravioli one at a time with a slotted spoon. Place a raviolo in each dish and spoon on the remaining butter. With a swivel-blade vegetable peeler, shave thin slices of the truffle, if using, or flakes of Parmigiano over the top. Serve immediately.

# *Beet Ravioli with Poppy Seeds*

## *Casunziei di Barbabietole Rosse*

**Makes 8 servings**

*In the Veneto, it is traditional to serve these beautiful ravioli at Christmas. I love the way the red beet filling shows through the pasta like a delicate blush. These ravioli are typical of Cortina d'Ampezzo, a world famous ski resort in the Alpine northern part of the region. The poppy seeds in the sauce reflect the influence of nearby Austria. Poppy seeds lose their freshness quickly at warm room temperatures, so smell them to be sure they have not turned rancid. Store poppy seeds in a tightly sealed container in the refrigerator or freezer.*

4 medium beets, trimmed and scrubbed

½ cup whole or part-skim ricotta

1 cup freshly grated Parmigiano-Reggiano

2 tablespoons plain dry bread crumbs

Salt and freshly ground black pepper

1 pound Fresh Egg Pasta, rolled out and cut into 4-inch strips

8 tablespoons (1 stick) unsalted butter

1 tablespoon poppy seeds

**1.** Place the beets in a medium saucepan with cold water to cover. Bring to a simmer and cook until tender when pierced with a knife, about 30 minutes. Drain and let cool.

**2.** Peel the beets and cut them into chunks. Place them in a food processor and chop finely. Add the ricotta, $^1/_2$ cup of the Parmigiano-Reggiano, bread crumbs, and salt and pepper to taste. Process just until blended but still slightly coarse.

**3.** Prepare the pasta. Make and cook the ravioli as described in the recipe for Cheese Ravioli, Steps 2 to 6.

**4.** Meanwhile, melt the butter with the poppy seeds and a pinch of salt. Pour half the butter into a warm serving bowl. Transfer the ravioli to the bowl. Spoon the remaining sauce over the ravioli and sprinkle with the remaining $^1/_2$ cup of Parmigiano-Reggiano. Serve immediately.

## *Meat-Filled Pasta Rings in Cream Sauce*

### *Tortellini alla Panna*

**Makes 8 servings**

*According to a romantic legend, these ring-shaped pasta pockets were invented by a cook who spied on the goddess Venus in her bath. Inspired by her beauty, he created a pasta in the shape of her navel. Other versions of the story say that the beauty was Caterina di Medici. Whatever the inspiration behind them, these are wonderful served swimming in a rich meat or chicken broth or a simple cream or butter sauce. Anything more than that would be overkill.*

4 tablespoons unsalted butter

4 ounces boneless pork loin, cut into 1-inch cubes

4 ounces imported Italian prosciutto

4 ounces mortadella

1½ cups freshly grated Parmigiano-Reggiano

1 large egg

¼ teaspoon freshly ground nutmeg

1 pound Fresh Egg Pasta, rolled out and cut into 4-inch strips

1½ cups heavy or whipping cream

Salt

**1.** Melt 2 tablespoons of the butter in a small skillet over medium heat. Add the pork and cook, stirring occasionally, until cooked through, about 20 minutes. Let cool.

**2.** In a food processor or meat grinder, grind the pork, prosciutto, and mortadella until very fine. Transfer the meats to a bowl. Stir in 1 cup of the Parmigiano-Reggiano, egg, and nutmeg.

**3.** Line 2 or 3 large baking sheets with lint-free towels. Dust the towels with flour.

**4.** Prepare the pasta. Working with one piece at a time, keep the remainder covered.

**5.** Cut the pasta into 2-inch squares. Place about 1/2 teaspoon of the filling on each square. Fold the dough over the filling to form a triangle. Press the edges together firmly to seal. Work quickly so that the dough does not dry out.

**6.** Bring the two opposite points of the triangle together to form a circle. Pinch the ends to seal. Place the formed tortellino on a baking sheet while you prepare the remaining dough and filling in the same way.

**7.** Refrigerate the tortellini up to several hours or overnight, turning the pieces occasionally. (For longer storage, freeze them on the baking sheet 1 hour or until firm, then transfer them to heavy-duty plastic bags and store in the freezer up to one month. Do not thaw before cooking.)

**8.** To make the sauce, melt the remaining 2 tablespoons of the butter with the cream and a pinch of salt in a skillet large enough to hold all of the pasta. Bring to a simmer and cook 1 minute or until lightly thickened.

**9.** Bring at least 4 quarts of water to a boil in a large pot. Add the tortellini and salt to taste. Stir occasionally until the water returns to a boil. Reduce the heat so that the water is boiling gently. Cook 3 minutes or until slightly underdone. Drain well.

**10.** Pour the tortellini into the skillet with the cream and stir gently. Add the remaining 1/2 cup of Parmigiano-Reggiano and stir again. Serve immediately.

# *Potato Tortelli with Sausage Ragù*

## *Tortelli di Patate al Ragù di Salsiccia*

**Makes 6 to 8 servings**

*Mashed potatoes flavored with Parmigiano-Reggiano fill fresh pasta rings in southern Emilia-Romagna and northern Tuscany. Instead of squares, as in the Meat-Filled Pasta Rings in Cream Sauce recipe, these start out as circles of dough and are then shaped into rings. Serve them with a rich Sausage Ragù, or simply enjoy them with Butter and Sage Sauce.*

4 1/2 cups Sausage Ragù

3 medium boiling potatoes

2 tablespoons unsalted butter, at room temperature

1 cup freshly grated Parmigiano-Reggiano

1/8 teaspoon freshly grated nutmeg

Salt and freshly ground black pepper

1 pound Fresh Egg Pasta, rolled out and cut into 4-inch strips

1. Prepare the ragù. Then, place the whole potatoes in a pot with cold water to cover. Bring to a simmer and cook until the potatoes are tender when pierced with a knife, about 20 minutes. Drain and let cool.

2. Peel the potatoes and mash them with a ricer or food mill until smooth. Stir in the butter, $^1/_2$ cup of the cheese, the nutmeg, and salt and pepper to taste.

3. Sprinkle two baking sheets with flour.

4. Prepare the pasta. With a 2-inch round cookie or biscuit cutter, or a small glass, cut the dough into circles. Place a teaspoon of the filling on one side of each circle. Dip a fingertip in cool water and moisten the dough circle halfway around. Fold the dough over the filling to form a semicircle. Press the edges firmly together to seal. Gather the two corners of the dough and pinch them together. Place the tortelli on the prepared baking sheet. Repeat with the remaining dough and filling.

5. Cover and refrigerate, turning the pieces occasionally, up to 3 hours. (For longer storage, freeze the pasta on the baking sheets. Transfer to heavy-duty plastic bags. Seal tightly and freeze up to one month. Do not thaw before cooking.)

6. When ready to cook the tortelli, bring at least 4 quarts of water to a boil. Bring the sauce to a simmer. Add the pasta to the boiling water with salt to taste. Stir well. Cook over medium heat, stirring frequently, until the pasta is tender yet still firm to the bite.

7. Spoon some of the sauce into a heated serving bowl. Drain the pasta well and add it to the bowl. Top with the remaining sauce and 1/2 cup cheese. Serve immediately.

## *Potato Gnocchi*

### *Gnocchi di Patate con Ragù o al Sugo*

**Makes 6 servings**

*Roman trattorias often have daily specials. Thursdays are usually their day to serve potato gnocchi, though gnocchi are also made for the big Sunday lunch at mama's house when the whole family gets together.*

*The important thing to remember in making potato gnocchi is to handle them gently and never overwork the potatoes by putting them in a food processor or mixer. The moisture content of the potatoes will determine how much flour you need.*

*If you have any doubts about whether you have added enough flour to the dough, try this trick suggested to me by a clever chef. Make a test* gnòcco. *Pinch off a small piece of dough and cook it in a small saucepan of boiling water until it floats to the surface, then cook it 30 seconds more. Scoop it out of the water and taste it. The dumpling should hold its shape without being mushy or tough. If it is too soft, knead in more flour. If it is tough, it probably has too much flour already. Either start all over again or try cooking the gnocchi a little longer.*

4 cups Neapolitan Ragù or Fresh Tomato Sauce

1½ pounds baking potatoes

About 2 cups all-purpose flour

1 large egg yolk, beaten

Salt

**1.** Prepare the ragù or sauce. Then, place the potatoes in a large pot with cold water to cover. Cover the pot and bring to a simmer. Cook until the potatoes are tender when pierced with a knife, about 20 minutes. Dust two large baking sheets with flour.

**2.** While the potatoes are still warm, peel them and cut them into chunks. Mash the potatoes, using the smallest holes of a ricer or food mill, or by hand with a potato masher. Add the egg yolk and 2 teaspoons of salt. Stir in one cup of the flour just until blended. The dough will be stiff.

**3.** Scrape the potatoes onto a floured surface. Knead briefly, adding only enough flour so that the gnocchi will hold their shape when cooked but not so much that they become heavy. The dough should be slightly sticky.

4. Set the dough aside. Scrape the board to remove any dough scraps. Wash and dry your hands, then dust them with flour. Set out one or two large baking pans and dust them with flour.

5. Cut the dough into 8 pieces. Keeping the remaining dough covered, roll one piece into a long rope about $^3/_4$ inch thick. Cut the rope into $^1/_2$ inch-long nuggets.

6. To shape the dough, hold a fork in one hand with the tines pointed down. With the thumb of the other hand, roll each piece of dough over the back of the tines, pressing lightly to make ridges on one side and an indentation from your finger on the other. Let the gnocchi drop onto the prepared pans. The pieces should not touch. Repeat with the remaining dough.

7. Refrigerate the gnocchi until ready to cook. (Gnocchi can also be frozen. Place the baking sheets in the freezer for one hour or until firm. Put the gnocchi in a large heavy-duty plastic bag. Freeze up to one month. Do not thaw before cooking.)

8. Have ready a heated shallow serving bowl. Pour a thin layer of the hot sauce into the bowl.

9. To cook the gnocchi, bring a large pot of water to a boil. Add 2 tablespoons salt. Lower the heat so that the water boils gently. Drop the gnocchi into the water a few pieces at a time. Cook for

30 seconds after the gnocchi rise to the surface. Skim the gnocchi from the pot with a slotted spoon, draining the pieces well. Transfer to the serving bowl. Repeat with remaining gnocchi.

**10.** Toss the gnocchi with the sauce. Spoon on the remaining sauce; sprinkle with cheese. Serve hot.

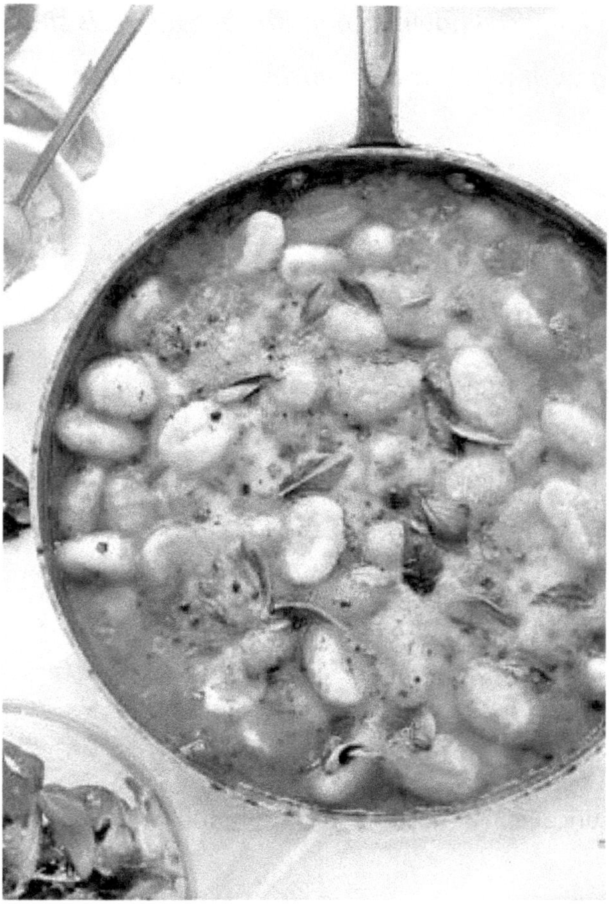

## *Potato Gnocchi with Lamb Ragù*

### *Gnocchi con Ragù di Agnello*

**Makes 6 to 8 servings**

*This recipe is from the Abruzzo region of central Italy. The sauce is typically served with pasta alla chitarra—homemade egg pasta cut with a special device known as a guitar because it is shaped like a frame strung with wires. It also works well in a hearty dish with gnocchi.*

1 pound Potato Gnocchi, through step 7

2 tablespoons olive oil

1 medium onion, finely chopped

1 red bell pepper, seeded and chopped

Pinch of crushed red pepper

2 garlic cloves, finely chopped

1 pound lean ground lamb

1 (28- to 35-ounce) can imported Italian tomatoes with their juice, chopped

1 tablespoon tomato paste

1 bay leaf

Salt to taste

½ cup freshly grated Pecorino Romano or Parmigiano-Reggiano

**1.** Prepare the gnocchi. Then, in a large skillet, cook the olive oil, onion, bell pepper, and red pepper until the vegetables are tender, about 10 minutes. Add the garlic and cook 1 minute more.

**2.** Stir in the lamb and cook 15 minutes, stirring frequently to break up any lumps, until it is no longer pink. Stir in the tomatoes. Add the tomato paste, bay leaf, and salt.

**3.** Bring the sauce to a simmer and reduce the heat to low. Cook, stirring occasionally, until the sauce is thickened, about 1½ hours.

**4.** Bring at least 4 quarts of water to a boil. Lower the heat so that the water boils gently. Drop the gnocchi into the water a few pieces at a time. Cook 30 seconds after the gnocchi rise to the surface.

**5.** Meanwhile, remove the bay leaf from the sauce. Spoon a thin layer into a large heated serving bowl. Skim the gnocchi from the pot with a slotted spoon, draining the pieces well. Add them to the bowl. Repeat with remaining gnocchi. Top with the remaining sauce and cheese. Serve hot.

# *Gratinéed Potato Gnocchi*

## *Gnocchi Gratinati*

**Makes 6 servings**

*In Piedmont, potato gnocchi are topped with cheese and bread crumbs and baked in a heat-proof oval dish known as a gratin. When baked, the cheeses melt and the crumbs become crunchy. The dish can be assembled ahead of time and baked just before you are ready to serve it.*

1 recipe Potato Gnocchi

2 tablespoons bread crumbs

Salt

6 ounces Fontina Valle d'Aosta

4 tablespoons unsalted butter

Freshly ground black pepper

¼ cup freshly grated Parmigiano-Reggiano

Pinch of cinnamon

1. Prepare the gnocchi. Then, place a rack in the center of the oven. Preheat the oven to 350°F. Butter a 13 × 9 × 2–inch baking dish. Sprinkle it with the breadcrumbs.

2. Bring a large pot of water to a boil. Add the gnocchi and salt to taste. Cook, stirring occasionally, for 30 seconds after the gnocchi float to the surface. Scoop out the gnocchi with a slotted spoon and make a layer of them in the prepared baking dish. Lay half of the Fontina on top and drizzle with half of the butter. Sprinkle with pepper. Make a second layer of gnocchi, Fontina and butter. Sprinkle with the grated cheese and cinnamon.

3. Bake 20 minutes or until bubbling and lightly golden. Serve hot.

# *Sorrento-Style Potato Gnocchi*

## *Gnocchi alla Sorrentina*

**Makes 8 servings**

*In the Naples area, potato gnocchi are often called strangolopreti, meaning "priest stranglers," the idea being that a greedy priest faced with such delicious home cooking might eat too many and choke. This baked dish is a specialty of Sorrento.*

About 2 cups Marinara Sauce

1 recipe Potato Gnocchi

Salt

8 ounces fresh mozzarella, thinly sliced

¼ cup freshly grated Pecorino Romano

**1.** Prepare the sauce and the gnocchi. Then, place a rack in the center of the oven. Preheat the oven to 400°F. Spread a thin layer of the sauce in a 13 × 9 × 2-inch baking dish.

**2.** Bring a large pot of water to a boil. Add salt to taste. Lower the heat so that the water boils gently. Drop the gnocchi into the water a few pieces at a time. Cook for 30 seconds after the gnocchi rise to the surface. Skim the gnocchi from the pot with a slotted spoon, draining the pieces well. Spread the gnocchi in the baking dish. Spoon on some of the sauce. Repeat with the remaining gnocchi and sauce. Scatter the mozzarella over the gnocchi. Sprinkle with the grated cheese.

**3.** Bake 30 minutes or until the sauce is bubbling. Serve hot.

CPSIA information can be obtained
at www.ICGtesting.com
Printed in the USA
LVHW020756270422
717291LV00014B/487

9 781804 506509